FITNESS OR FICTION

The **Truth** About Diet and Exercise

By
Brent **Brookbush**

MS, PES, CES, CSCS, ACSM-H/FS

ISBN: 0615503012
ISBN-13: 9780615503011

Table of Contents

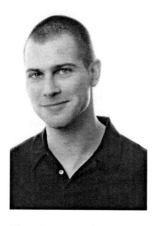

Brent Brookbush,
MS, PES, CES, CSCS, ACSM-H/FS
President, B2C Fitness, LLC –
Integrated Education System

Experience: Since 1998 Brent has educated 1000's of personal trainers, written and consulted for various fitness magazines, and has been a revered personal trainer. Passionate about changing lives and focused on delivering evidence based practical education Brent has been a resource for industry giants like, New York Sports Clubs, Equinox, NASM, HFPN, SHAPE Magazine, and Power Plate. As president of B2C Fitness, he continues to develop cutting-edge training and development systems and educational publications for fitness professionals. Currently Brent is an Instructor for PowerPlate, NASM, and B2C Fitness, and is grateful for the opportunity to impact the lives of 100's of personal trainers each year.

Degrees:
Bachelor of Science: Health and Wellness: Sports Management, California University of Pennsylvania
Master of Science: Exercise Science: Focus in Rehabilitation Science, California University of Pennsylvania
Doctoral Student at CUNY/Hunter - Graduate Center, Clinical Doctorate of Physical Therapy program.

Certifications:
NASM – Certified Personal Trainer
          Integrated Flexibility Specialist
          Performance Enhancement Specialist
          Corrective Exercise Specialist
NSCA – Certified Personal Trainer
          Certified Strength and Conditioning Specialist
ACSM – Health/Fitness Specialist
NFPT – Certified Fitness Trainer
NHE – Certified Master Trainer
FMS – Certified Specialist

Introduction:

The fitness industry is an anomaly. In no other health field would we allow the popular media to dictate the practice of professionals. In no other health field is the information from the Internet, newspapers, and TV considered more accurate than information from governing bodies and credentialed professionals.

The fitness industry is unregulated and profit driven. It is like a journalist who wrote about heart medication, received a kickback from that medication, and then started prescribing that medication to everyone. Or, a marathon runner who could start practicing as a cardiologist because of his excellent cardiovascular conditioning. Prescribing medication and monitoring the heart requires a physician – a credentialed, formally educated professional, and you should expect nothing less from the fitness industry.

Yet within the fitness industry, it is commonplace to accept advice from "gurus" who lack any formal education, credentials, or training. These "gurus" rely on a fit body and guesswork to promote kooky products and ideas. But, a fit body is not a reflection of someone's fitness knowledge, and there is no need for guesswork. Getting and staying fit is a science that has been developing for decades. Science and research is progressing faster than ever, and there are credentialed professionals working hard to make this information available to you.

As an educator for the largest health club chains on the east coast, I have trained thousands of individuals just like you not only to get fit, but to become personal trainers themselves. I understand how to make the science and research of fitness practical, and can help you apply the same cutting-edge techniques used by the pros. I know what fitness trends have merit and which ones are bogus. I can teach you what I teach certified professionals, making your goals more attainable than ever before.

Examples:

You cannot tone, but you can choose exercises that will burn more calories and lead to a leaner physique.

You cannot eat more, move less, and lose weight, but weight loss can be accomplished with the foods and activity you enjoy.

You cannot focus on details and expect big picture change, but understanding the big picture will make big change simpler than ever before.

If you keep doing the same things you will continue to look the same way. It's time to make a change. There are no secrets, no tricks, and no one is hiding the answer from you. With the information in this book, you can steer clear of gimmicks and create your own personalized fitness program. No more misleading diet plans and products that promise unattainable results. You can be your own personal trainer and critically evaluate your options. You can use the equipment that is available to you now, or enter the fitness market with the information you need to make the right decision. Stop <u>fighting</u> your body and start <u>working with</u> your body.

Special Thanks:

This book is my attempt to a fill a void in fitness. A means of bridging the gap between the brightest minds in health and wellness and those pursuing a healthy lifestyle - An attempt to explain health science in simple English without the bias of sponsorship, product placement, and profits. However, I must admit there have been outside influences. *There is no way I could have written this book without the help, mentorship, and friendship of some incredibly talented people.*

Thanks to Rick Richey for being the inspiration that launched my career in fitness education. Your insights, mentorship, support, and friendship have been a gift. Your talent continues to be an inspiration and I look forward to the change we can make in the fitness industry. Thanks to Doug Hatten for taking a chance and giving me my first teaching opportunity. Your continued mentorship has been instrumental in my development and growth, and I have no doubt that you will continue to be instrumental in my career. Thank you to my editors, Sabila Kahn and Rakia Clark. You have developed a poor English student into an author – no easy task. Thank you to my friends at SHAPE magazine - Trisha Calvo, Janet Lee, and John Balen. Your continued support and enlightening conversations were instrumental in shaping the voice of this book. Thank you to my friend and fantastic photographer Gorgia Nerheim for the photography and to Definitions – Private Training Gyms for giving us a wonderful place to take the photographs.

Thank you, thank you, thank you for helping me to communicate a message. I could not have come this far without you. Much, much love…

SECTION I:
THE BASICS

Chapter 1:
Food, Calories, and Diets

Nutrition may be the most misunderstood topic in the fitness industry. More than $30 billion is spent on weight loss strategies per year, most of this money spent on diet products[98]. Yet we continue to get fatter, suffer from preventable disease, and succumb to the social stigmas and psychological pressures that excess weight and poor health bring upon us.

The cause of our problem is not a lack of information. The problem in the fitness industry is *too much* information; that is, too much contradicting information. Studies have shown that even Division 1 college athletes have a poor understanding of nutrition; most of the athletes acquiring their information from questionable sources, such as magazines, family members, and coaches who have a limited understanding of nutrition themselves[74-76].

Ahead are common myths debunked and the answer to the nutrition questions that concern you. Learning the truth can help you find simple solutions that will improve your eating habits.

Myth #1: *Anybody who has the title of "Doctor" must know something about nutrition.*
What You Should Know: Doctors are not nutritionists.

This is one of my biggest pet-peeves. I started college as a jazz studies major, and if things had worked out differently, I would have gone on to acquire my Ph.D. in music. A Ph.D. gives me the title of doctor, but like a medical doctorate it would not provide me with the education I needed to be an expert in nutrition.

Are you aware that most medical doctors are only required to take one, maybe two semesters of nutrition. Yet, medical doctors who specialize in oncology, cardiology, or even podiatry pass themselves off as experts in nutrition. Nutritionists spend years studying various nutrients and how they affect the body's systems -- not a semester or two. They dedicate their lives to enhancing the health of individuals through better nutrition practices. Many states require registered dieticians to acquire an M.S. in nutrition, participate in a six month internship, and pass a state licensure exam before they can begin to practice. The knowledge a nutritionist acquires about eating is far more extensive than the knowledge acquired by a medical doctor. I do not take issue with health professionals educating the public on general nutrition practices. However, it is misleading for M.D.s to advertise themselves as nutrition experts. Put bluntly, M.D.'s need to stay in their lane. I am surprised there is not a class action lawsuit against some of these doctors for a breach of scope.

Myth #2: *Carbohydrates are your enemy.*
What You Should Know: Excess calories are your enemy, not carbs!

Carbohydrates have a very important role in the human body. They are your most important source of energy - "your master fuel." Anaerobic activities like sprinting, lifting, and sport rely on sugar for fuel; fat simply cannot be broken down fast enough to fuel high intensity activities. When fat does provide a large percentage of your energy, carbohydrates are needed to start the process that burns fat. In this way even fat burns in a carbohydrate flame. Carbohydrates are also the primary energy source for the nervous system. The nervous system relies on sugar in the blood stream to meet its energy needs. When blood sugar levels fall the nervous system suffers. You may have been witness to a diabetic suffering from a blood sugar crash and the immediate effect such a crash has on their nervous system - confusion, clumsiness, and disorientation.

Carbohydrates in moderation are essential to a healthy diet. Whether it is a sugar, a starch, simple, complex, bread, pasta, potato, fruit, or vegetable, carbohydrates are vital to the normal function of our bodies. Carbohydrates should be the source of 45-65% of your daily calories[52]. Many sources of complex carbohydrates are also vital in supplying us with the vitamins, minerals and fiber we need. (For potential risks of a low carb diets see Ketogenic Diets later in this chapter). So carbs are good!!!

What is bad? It's simple. Consuming more calories than we burn is bad. This is a very important concept that fitness and diet gurus have tried to skirt around for years. All food we eat and drink provides us with calories, which are little units of energy. Energy cannot be created or destroyed, only transferred or changed from one form to another (First law of thermodynamics).

If *excess* calories are consumed, they cannot be destroyed. They must be transferred, and if not immediately needed for energy or metabolic functions, the excess energy will likely be stored as fat. This means that no matter what you eat, if energy input is more than energy output, you will gain weight. Heck, you could gain weight eating lettuce. It would take a whole lot of lettuce, but if you eat enough, the result will be the same. If you understand this concept there is little if any mystery behind weight loss. It is all math.

Example:

Let's say I am a weight-stable individual. That is, I have not gained or lost any weight recently. We can assume that my "calories consumed" are equal to my "calories burned". If I increased what I ate by 500 calories a day and decreased my physical activity so that I burned 500 calories less a day, I would end up with a 1000 calorie per day surplus. One week would amount to a 7000 calorie surplus. One pound of stored fat is approximately 3500 stored calories. So at the end of one week I would end up with two extra pounds of body fat.

- 500 extra calories consumed + 500 calories not burned = 1000 extra calories per day
- 1000 calories x 7 days in a week = 7000 calories extra per week

- Excess calories are generally stored as fat, and 1 pound of fat is roughly 3500 stored calories.
- 7000 divided by 3500 = 2 pounds

Consuming more calories than I burn is an all too common scenario during the holidays. Because of various parties, dinners, and travel to see my family, I often miss my daily workout, which reduces my daily energy expenditure. We all know how easy it is to take in extra calories during the holidays. Five hundred calories would be equivalent to a glass of red wine and a moderate-sized dessert. If you multiply the 2 pounds per week by the number of weeks between Thanksgiving and New Year's it is easy to see how one can put on 10 or even 15 pounds during the holidays.

Ketogenic Diets: To Carb, or Not to Carb?

Ketogenic diets are those diets that emphasize carbohydrate restrictions while generally ignoring the total caloric content of the diet. Although these diets may be effective for losing a quick ten pounds (primarily due to relative dehydration) they have not been shown to be any more effective than a standard well-balanced diet at lowering body fat[3]. The health concerns far outweigh the potential benefit of the weight loss on these diets, and there is much concern for long term compliance.

If you are a man or woman who maintains a physically active lifestyle, your diet should be 45% to 65% carbohydrates. Most of your carbohydrates sources should be in the form of starches, fiber-rich unprocessed grains, fruits, and vegetables[52]. Even The Zone diet which is 40% carbs has been shown to reduce exercise performance[79]. Although advocates of low carb diets will claim that you are burning more fat; this is not the case. On a normal diet, a well nourished individual uses primarily fat to fuel metabolic functions at rest[52].

Many people will sacrifice a healthful diet and the enjoyment of many foods to shed a couple of extra pounds. Vegetables, fruits, whole grains, potatoes, and cereal are all rich in carbohydrates, and are good examples of foods you should be eating. They're staples of a healthy diet. Subscribing to a low-carb diet is not only restrictive and ineffective for long-term weight loss; it can be dangerous. Consider the potential risks below.

Potential Risks of Low Carb Diets:

Ketoacidosis: The breakdown of fat and protein in the absence of carbohydrates produces ketone bodies. Supporters claim that these ketone bodies suppress appetite, and ketones lost in the urine represent lost energy. However, this lost energy is likely not significant enough to be an effective method of weight loss. It is far more likely that ketone bodies could create a potentially dangerous state of acidity within the body known as ketosis. Further, if left unchecked, ketosis could lead to a clinical condition known as ketoacidosis, eventually coma, and possibly even death[52]. It is estimated that roughly 50 to 100 grams (200 to 400 calories worth) of carbohydrates per day is needed to prevent ketosis[9].

Reduced functioning and/or damage to your nervous system: Blood sugar levels must be maintained within a very narrow margin to ensure that there is enough circulating blood sugar for your nervous system. When the liver has to rely on the breakdown of protein to provide sugar to the central nervous system, it becomes difficult for your body to maintain blood sugar levels within this narrow margin. When blood sugar levels drop, symptoms may include weakness, dizziness, and impaired exercise performance. Extreme levels of low blood sugar can cause a loss of consciousness and irreversible brain damage. You may have witnessed the disorientation and lack of coordination experienced by diabetics during a blood sugar crash[52].

Loss of Muscle: Low carbohydrate diets can lead to a significant loss of lean tissue. Your body will start recruiting protein in muscle tissue to maintain blood sugar if sufficient carbohydrates are not present. This may actually cause a protein deficiency, even when a person ingests protein well above the norm[52]. Adequate carbohydrate intake helps to preserve tissue proteins by ensuring that carbohydrates are used for your energy needs and protein is left to be used for tissue repair, growth, and maintenance.

Note: Each kilogram (2.2 pounds) of muscle burns approximately 77 calories per day. With each pound of muscle lost, your metabolism may slow. This could have a very negative effect on your long term weight loss goals, and the lost muscle will make it tougher to keep a "toned" appearance.

Risk of Osteoporosis: Ketogenic diets may increase the risk for osteoporosis. Two factors that contribute to osteoporosis are a lack of calcium, and bone mineral loss[9]. Calcium and bone minerals act to buffer acidity in the body, such as the ketosis mentioned above. It is estimated that with every gram of protein consumed *above that needed for tissue maintenance*, between 1 and 1.5 grams of calcium is excreted as well[2]. In low-carb diets, protein is usually ingested in much larger amounts than is recommended.

High fat diets contribute to the risk of various diseases: Often individuals on low-carb diets ingest high levels of fat. High amounts of fat in the diet may constitute a risk for heart disease and diabetes, as well as several cancers, including ovarian, colon, and breast cancer[2-5]. Elevation in serum cholesterol eventually produces a degenerative process known as arteriosclerosis, or a hardening and narrowing of medium and large sized arteries[2-5]. Fat intake should not exceed 30% of one's diet, and 70%-80% of that should be split between mono-**un**saturated and poly**un**saturated fats[2-5]. Cholesterol should also be limited to less than 300mg per day[2-5].

Excess fat is easy to convert into body fat: The body is particularly efficient at converting excess calories of dietary fat into stored fat[7]. Consequently, greater increases in body fat can occur when the diet is high in fat content compared to an equivalent caloric excess of carbohydrates.

Fatigue and reduced performance during exercise and sport: Carbohydrates are a chief source of energy for all bodily functions and muscular exertion. Several studies have shown a decrease in performance while on ketogenic or high fat diets[9, 30, 96, 134]. In one study a diet high in fat with less than 5% carbohydrates reduced muscle glycogen (sugar) by 64%[96]. In similar studies high fat diets have shown that a reduction in muscle glycogen will result in fatigue, and reduce endurance capacity by half during cardiovascular exercise (treadmill, bike) when compared to a normal diet[9, 30]. Low carbohydrate diets also have similar effects on intense short term exercise, such as weight lifting[9, 30].

Dehydration: The dehydration associated with ketogenic diets is caused by two primary factors.

The digestion, metabolization, and excretion of protein and its byproducts, and depletion of glycogen stores and the subsequent water stored with them. (The depletion of glycogen and water loss is discussed below under "What's up with these crash diets?"

It takes a significant amount of water to digest protein and rid the body of byproducts associated with protein and fat metabolism (ketone bodies, and nitrogen) when carbohydrates are restricted or absent from the diet[52]. Your body rids itself of these byproducts by excreting them in your urine, but they must first be diluted in water. The decrease in stored water and dehydration from protein metabolism and excretion of byproducts is likely the cause of the rapid reduction in weight with little or no reduction in body fat[148].

Nutrient Deficiency: Foods categorized as complex carbohydrates generally have high nutrient densities, which means they carry large amounts of vitamins and minerals your body needs. Without them, nutrient deficiencies can occur[5, 52].

Altered Electrolyte levels: Ketogenic diets may alter electrolyte levels (major electrolytes are sodium, potassium, chloride, magnesium, and calcium) causing undesirable heart arrhythmias (fluctuation in heart beat)[52].

Do not follow a low carb diet during pregnancy: Carbohydrates are essential to fetal development. This diet is contraindicated during pregnancy[52].

Interesting Tidbits: At the turn of the twentieth century carbohydrate intake, as a percentage of total calories, was higher, fat as a percentage was lower, and obesity was not the problem it is today[30]. Currently, total fat intake is higher, carbohydrate intake is lower, and obesity has reached epidemic proportions[30]. Know that America's problem with obesity is not a direct result of carbo-hydrate consumption, it is the result of a too many calories and not enough activity.

Myth #3: *You can lose eight pounds of fat in a week.*
What You Should Know: The eight pounds is not fat.

Often diets promote rapid weight loss, with marketing slogans like "lose 10 pounds in 2 weeks", or "I lost eight pounds the first week I was on the _____ diet." Note that the ads state weight loss and not fat loss. Rapid weight loss is neither healthy nor safe and does not usually result in large amounts of fat loss. In fact, losing eight to ten pounds of fat in a week would be nearly impossible. The weight lost during crash diets and low carb diets can be attributed to the depletion of muscle glycogen, relative dehydration, and the breakdown of proteins in muscle (muscle loss) and liver.

Why does this dehydration and muscle loss occur rather than burning the fat I want to lose?
It all comes down to sugar (carbs). Your body cannot live without it. If you do not consume enough carbs, your body has to find a way to make sugar. The steps below summarize this process.

Step 1: *Your body depletes stored sugar (glycogen) from your body*

- When you eat enough carbs (whether simple or complex) they fuel activity and help to replenish the sugar stored within your muscles that is utilized during your day. If inadequate amounts are consumed your body will deplete sugar stores and quickly.

Step 2: *Water and sugar are stored together within muscle and liver tissue. The depletion of sugar leads to a loss of total body water:*

- Unfortunately no amount of water is going to make up for this relative dehydration. You can drink a gallon of water per day,

10

but your body cannot retain it. It's like pouring water into a paper cup with a hole in the bottom. You can fill that cup over and over, but until you plug the hole (take in more carbs) you cannot fill the cup. Such water loss has no lasting significance in a program designed to reduce body fat. The weight is likely to return when carbohydrates are ingested and the body's water balance returns to normal[30]. Keep in mind dehydration puts serious strain on many systems within in the body.

Step 3: *Your body must turn to protein to create more sugar.*

- Your body cannot make enough sugar, quickly enough, from fat. So it turns to protein to fill the gap. One of your body's largest protein reserves is your muscle tissue. Until an adequate amount of carbohydrates is returned to your diet, your body will continue to break down muscle tissue. Remember that muscle is important for your metabolism, your toned appearance, and most importantly, your daily functions. No amount of resistance training or increase in protein consumption is going to offset the unfortunate consequences of relying on protein as a primary fuel source.

Step 4: *Fatigue*

- At the very least, a diet extremely low in calories or carbohydrates is going to result in fatigue. These diets force your body to use more complex and less efficient means of producing sugar, and your body does not like to run this way. Studies show rapid weight loss decreases performance[136]. So in the end, you are not only losing the wrong type of weight, but your workouts that will promote the right type of weight loss (fat loss) are less than optimal, which in turn reduces the amount of calories you burn.

Rapid weight loss from crash and low-carb diets is only temporary. As soon as you return to a normal, healthful diet that includes carbohydrates, the water weight will return and glycogen stores will be replenished. So, while the result of your crash diet and "sugar storage" depletion is rapid weight loss, you lost very little fat, and will likely have very little long-term change.

Anytime someone has told me a fantastical story of rapid weight loss I have to ask myself, "What would it take to burn eight pounds of fat in a week?" "Is it possible to lose 8 pounds a week in a healthy way?"

To lose eight pounds of fat you would have to create a caloric deficit of 28,000 calories (3500 x 8). If you ate 1000 calories less per day you could lose two pounds, leaving just 21000 calories to burn. According to ACSM's metabolic equation for running, a person weighing 150 pounds running at 6.0 miles per hour would have to run for 30.17 hours or 181 miles to burn that many calories[71]. That's equivalent to running a marathon every day for a week!!! If you want to burn eight pounds of fat in a week, it would require an extreme caloric restriction and nearly nonstop moderate intensity activity. Not healthy, not admirable, and likely impossible.

When faced with this evidence the response to any question regarding rapid weight loss is usually replaced with admiration for the steady 1-2 pounds of fat loss per week. Although this is not easy to hear for some, one to two pounds a week still results in 50 to 100 pounds of weight loss in just one year.

Myth #4: *Fat is your enemy.*
What You Should Know: Once again, excess calories from *any* source are your enemy.

If people are not scared of carbohydrates than they are scared of fat. But fat is essential to keeping you alive and should make up 20-35% of your total calories[5, 52]. In two very interesting studies, highly trained competitive cyclists were asked to eat a *calorie controlled* diet high in fat (42% and 50% of total calories). Yet, the increase in fat content of the diet did not cause weight gain or increase risk factors associated with heart disease[23, 92]. The details to note in this study are the high level of activity of the participants and that despite an increase in fat, the total calories of the diet stayed the same.

Fat is an important source of energy, and stored body fat serves as our most abundant energy reserve. Stored fat provides protection for vital organs, and acts as a thermal and electrical insulator in the body. Fat acts as a carrier for various substances in the body including fat soluble vitamins A, D, E, and K, and the fat in food helps to contribute to satiety (the feeling of being full) which can be beneficial for those on a diet.

Although the fear of fat is an unnecessary phobia, I can understand the rationale behind it. Fat packs a lot of calories into a very small package, making it easy to consume too many calories. I would assume that in the studies mentioned above; the increase in fat as a percentage of total calories reduced the total volume of food the cyclists were allowed to consume. Compare popular brands of peanut butter with steamed spinach - 100 calories per tablespoon versus 100 calories per 2 ½ cups. Saturated and trans fats are also potentially dangerous, and have been linked to an increase risk of heart disease[5].

Don't run from fat; but minimize the amount of fried foods, deserts, and butter you use. All things in moderation! Less than 10% of the fat in your diet should be in the form of saturated and/or trans-fats[5].

Myth #5: *I have fat parents so I am destined to be fat.*
What You Should Know: You are in control of your weight.

This myth implies that both genetics and the behaviors we learn from our parents determine our future fatness. Studies have shown that as many obese children come from two normal weight parents as children who have two obese parents[10, 165]. The truth is genetics may play a role in obesity and excess weight, by as much as 25-40 percent[10]. But the jury is still out. No research relieves responsibility from an overweight population. Those who are overweight must make healthier choices and take responsibility for poor choices.

One recent study attempted to correlate the athletic ability of adolescents and obesity. It examined how efficiently overweight children and normal weight children move during exercise and compared the resting metabolism of overweight children and their normal weight peers. No link could be made[165]; implying that overweight children start with the same athletic ability and metabolism as their thinner counterparts. Studies, however, have made a startling connection between poor youth fitness and adult fatness[147, 168]. In the end, the factors we can control are activity, eating habits, and education. Find activities you enjoy and learn the skills that will make you better at them, learn about healthy food choices and find food you enjoy, and when possible start learning those habits young.

Myth #6: *I have a slow metabolism.*
What You Should Know: This may be an "Old Wives' Tale."

I have yet to see research comparing the metabolism of individuals of the same size and activity level. That leaves this myth open to debate. However, I believe it is far more likely that individuals who claim to have a fast metabolism are probably, younger, more active, are larger (not fatter, but physically larger), have more muscle, and/or eat less than their counterparts with a "slower metabolism."

Myth #7: *You can't eat that!*
What You Should Know: You can eat that!

"There is no such thing as a bad food. Everything is okay in moderation." Ever used this line before? Well it is true. Any food that does not surpass your energy needs or disrupt your nutrient balance can be added into a balanced diet. The trick is understanding moderation. Even pizza can be a lunch option if you settle for a slice and eat moderately throughout the day. A piece of cheesecake may be a great reward for a week when you accomplish all your fitness goals. The trouble lies in those who "cheat" almost daily, and continually create a caloric surplus in their diet. This is an important diet tip. Stay dedicated, but don't push yourself so hard that the craving eats away at you. Slowly, your little want becomes a little need then a little obsession and finally a fatal attraction. Over time all you think about is a burger and fries. They seem to have more value than gold and diamonds. You drool every time you pass the Fat Burger that those maniacal bastards put next door to the gym. Then one day in the middle of your umpteenth set of squats, you can't stand it. You flip out, kick your trainer, give the front desk the finger, run to Fat Burger, order enough food to graze on for two hours, only to realize you left your stuff at the gym, and have to walk back with a milkshake in your hand, ketchup on your face, and guilt in your eyes.

Myth #8: *If you eat before you go to bed you will gain weight.*
What You Should Know: Weight gain is not a scheduled event.

I believe the origin of this myth is the weight loss some people have experience by cutting out any source of calories after dinner. In essence, no dessert. Although this is a great tip for those trying to lose weight, it is the reduction in calories that causes the weight loss, not the time those calories were restricted.

Let's say I burn 2000 calories a day, but the only thing I ate one day is a pint of Ben and Jerry's (1300 calories, don't ask me how I know) before going to bed. I would lose weight. I'm at a 700 calorie deficit!!! Sure, the majority of that particular meal may be stored as fat, but I was burning fat (my stored energy) to stay alive all day. I would still wake up the next morning 700 calories lighter than the day before.

Note: Nobody get any bright ideas and try the above example. I am not suggesting a new diet plan, "The Ben Jerry's Diet"; this diet would be very unhealthy, and if done regularly would make you feel awful… It might be fun for a day, but absolutely unhealthy.

Myth #9: *There is a mysterious science behind weight loss that only trainers and their star clients know.*
What You Should Know: There is science, but no mystery.

Whether a person eats less, works more, or both, total calories ingested must be less than that burned if you wish to lose the fat. Put bluntly, Shut your face, and move your ass! If more energy is spent than ingested, your body must find a way to fuel activity. This is what your fat stores are for. Think of fat as stored, or potential, energy. If you wake up, look in the mirror and see more "potential energy" than you would like, find a way to use it.

Any diet, supplement, prescription drug, or piece of fad exercise equipment that is successful in reducing weight works because it creates a caloric deficit in one way or another that inevitably leads to weight loss. For someone to say that weight loss happens any other way (save fluctuations in water weight) is on par with someone trying to levitate to spite the laws of gravity. Both ideas defy the laws of physics.

So what is the suggested reduction in calories and increase in exercise for someone who wishes to lose weight? In a position statement by the American College of Sports Medicine, it was recommended that an energy deficit of 500 - 1000 calories per day is reached by restricting the amount of calories you eat. It is also recommend that overweight individuals gradually increase their physical activity to 2.5 hours per week at a moderate intensity. In time, one may consider increasing his or her workout to 3.5 to 5 hours per week, and upping the intensity[3, 73]. This should result in a loss of one to two pounds per week, which is healthy and easier to maintain. Think of how you could look in just one year.

How much weight can I lose per week?

For ideal, long-term benefits, it is recommended that 1 to 2 pounds or 1% of bodyweight is lost per week[9, 52, 71]. A pound of fat is 3500 stored calories, so, to lose 1-2 pounds takes a caloric deficit of 3500-7000 calories, and significant effort. I know this is not easy to hear for the many of us who have been sold by fad diets and gimmicks claiming 5-8 pounds per week. But, gradual weight loss ensures maximum fat loss and preservation of lean tissue. Remember that more lean tissue means a faster metabolism. In fact, rapid weight loss can result in the loss of three times more lean tissue than fat tissue[9]. This would have a very serious affect on your metabolism and may even hinder long-term weight loss goals.

How do I figure out how many calories I need?

Numerous variables effect your caloric requirements, making it difficult to use formulas or standardized numbers to calculate the amount of calories you need (although there are plenty of formulas out there.) Variables that change your caloric requirements include size, age, sex, and activity level, amount of muscle, temperature, environment and caloric intake[52].

The easiest way to monitor your caloric intake and make the necessary adjustments is to monitor your bodyweight[30]. If your weight has not changed over time you can assume that you are consuming as many calories as you burn per day. If you have been steadily gaining weight you are consuming more calories than you burn. If you have lost weight over time you are consuming less calories than you burn. Adjust your caloric intake and activity level according to your fitness goals, and continue to monitor your body weight.

Note: Your weight may change drastically by 1 to 4 pounds over the course of a day or a week. This is likely due to changes in hydration. Monitor weight often, but judge over weeks.

Myth #10: *Diet alone is the best way to lose weight.*
What You Should Know: Exercise is still the single best predictor of long-term success for those trying to lose weight[17].

But, less than half of those individuals trying to lose weight use exercise as part of their program, and less than half of the exercising individuals meet the recommended guidelines[172]. This may be a contributing factor to why so many individuals fail to reach their weight loss goals. Diet combined with exercise is more effective than either behavior alone, and it drastically increases health benefits, including a reduction in risk of coronary heart disease, diabetes, osteoporosis, and obesity[17, 77-78, 145]. Resistance training, cardio, and a flexibility program make wonderful additions to a healthy lifestyle and are covered in depth in the following chapters.

Note: Exercise does not have to be done at a gym. Daily activities, like walking to work, walking to lunch, gardening, housework, or even taking the stairs instead of the elevator all count towards your daily physical activity.

Positive effects of exercise while dieting:
1. Individuals who increase physical activity usually do not increase their caloric intake to match the new amount of calories their burning[19]. This could help tip the scales in favor of weight loss.
2. Long-term restrictive diets may affect the performance of your immune system resulting in more colds, and flu's. Exercise reduces the effects diet can have on immune function[128].
3. Exercise prevents the reduction in muscle mass usually found with diet alone[3, 71, 85]. Keep in mind that increasing muscle mass has a profound effect on resting metabolism. The more muscle mass you have, the more calories you burn.
4. Exercise promotes fat utilization for fueling activity[15]. More fat burned means less fat stored.
5. Exercise also decreases the amount of protein used for fuel, allowing protein to be used for muscle repair and growth[43].
6. In a treadmill test, resistance training of leg musculature increased muscular endurance. This implies that resistance training may allow you to train longer during your cardio endeavors and burn more calories[90].

More on Myth# 10: Some diet tips to help you with your weight loss efforts.

Be patient: For ideal long-term benefits, it is recommended that one to two pounds, or one percent of bodyweight, is lost per week. Gradual weight loss ensures maximum fat loss and preservation of muscle. Avoid extremely restrictive and/or crash diets, and stay focused on long-term changes.

Don't drink your calories: Just because you drink it does not mean it is calorie-free. Soda, fruit juice, and alcoholic beverages are diet sabotage. In a weight loss program, every calorie you consume from beverages must be subtracted from the food you eat. This can only add to hunger pains. Not to mention, the nutrient density of soda, alcoholic beverages, and most fruit juices is relatively low.

Spacing your meals evenly throughout the day could help to reduce hunger pains and grazing: Many of my clients skip meals or do not eat while at work. This usually results in grazing from the time they get home to the time they go to bed. Although hunger is natural when on a weight-loss program, starving yourself could lead to snacking and grazing which may result in consuming excess calories. Try to refrain from snacking and time your three meals so that hunger is only noted shortly before your next meal.

Keep a "Food Log": Many studies have shown that eating habits change when a person is held accountable to a written contract. A food log will force you to reflect on the food you have eaten, note the mistakes you have made, and show some forethought in your food choices. Also, you may find it easier to make adjustments in your diet when you are able to see the habits you have. Examples: Keep a healthy snack on hand for your favorite cheat times, or plan better meals for times when you are routinely bad, such as lunch at work.

Portion control: The easiest way to reduce your calories is to reduce your portion size at meals. All fat loss occurs because of a caloric deficit. Try a smaller bowl of cereal in the morning, half a sandwich for lunch, using a smaller plate at dinner, or reducing the amount of soda and fruit juice you drink.

Fat attack: Stay away from high-fat foods. Although fat is not your enemy, it is calorically dense. This is the reason why fast food can be so devastating to your weight loss efforts. A relatively small amount of food can pack a large amount of calories. It's just not worth it.

Just stop snacking: Even small snacks consumed throughout the day can add a significant amount of calories. One hundred excess calories per day would cause a gain of almost a pound a month, and 10 pounds in a year!!!

No more midnight munchies: Although eating before you go to bed will not cause weight gain by itself, cutting out snacks after dinner would help to reduce your caloric intake.

Pace yourself when drinking: Alcohol has a whopping seven calories per gram. Compare that to the four calories per gram in protein and carbohydrates and you can come to the quick conclusion that alcohol can pack on the pounds. The trick I use to curb my consumption is to have a glass of water between each alcoholic beverage. This slows down my pace and has the added effect of keeping me well-hydrated. Note: Dehydration is one of the factors that contribute to the dreaded hangover.

Stay away from adding sugar to your beverages: Many of us have become addicted to our morning cup of coffee (me included), but the sugar you add can really add up. This is especially true if you are hooked on the sweeter things on your coffee shop menu. Stay away from anything that has added syrup or chocolate.

Variety is the spice of life: Eat a variety of nutrient-dense foods to ensure that you are receiving all the vitamins and minerals you need. Try new things in your produce section or make it a habit to eat fish a couple times a week. Maybe you should try different carbohydrate sources like okra, sweet potatoes, or a three bean soup.

Water wise: Obviously, water is essential to our daily life, but how much do we actually need? Two to three liters of water per day for the average individual is good.

Extremely active individuals and larger individuals may require more. Dehydration impairs almost every physiological function. More water could mean better workouts, and better workouts could yield larger results. More water may also contribute to satiety, reducing your hunger pains.

Impact carbs have no impact on fat loss: One of the latest trends in our quick-fix society is the "impact carb" or "net carb count." This is just a gimmick to sell another product on the "low carb diet" band wagon. These low carb foods (generally in the form of bars) use sugar alcohol instead of simple sugars to hide the fact that they still pack the same amount of calories. Regardless of their effect on immediate insulin response, if these calories are not needed for immediate energy, these grams of sugar alcohol will also be stored as fat.

Label awareness: Most of the products we consume have the amount of calories listed right on the label, but have you ever paid close attention to the serving size? Sometimes it's the little things that get the best of us. Many products we consume and enjoy on a regular basis have misleading food labels. Companies will list the calories per serving, but list several servings per "package." For example, I was looking at a popular sports drink the other day that had just 90 calories per serving. The catch was that each 16oz bottle contained 2.5 serving. I actually consumed 225 calories.

Soup or salad: Salads, save the dressing, have a ton of vitamins and minerals and fewer calories per volume. You get more "bang for your buck." You can eat a lot of salad and take in a relatively small amount of calories, where as a burger may have twice as many calories and be a quarter of the size. Soups work in a similar fashion.

Myth #11: *I work-out, so I don't need to watch what I eat.*
What You Should Know: We are far more efficient at consuming calories than we are at burning them.

Although you may never hear the statement, "I workout, so I can eat whatever I want," you will often see this behavior. People often reward their exercise efforts with foods that are calorically dense, or they indulge in an excessively large meal. Sometimes they give themselves an all out cheat day. Some individuals workout hard, hope that's enough, and do not change their eating habits at all. If your goal is weight loss, you need to make changes to both your activity level and the amount of calories you ingest.

You can burn between 300 and 800 calories per hour during a work-out (depending on your size and intensity), but you can consume this many calories, and more, in 5 minutes or less, with a burger, fries, and a coke. I am not saying that you cannot cheat on occasion, just refrain from making it a habit.

Myth #12: *Lifting heavy things will make your muscles bigger.*
What you should know: Lifting alone won't do it.

For those individuals who wish not only to gain muscle mass, but weight as well, a combination of diet and progressive resistance training is essential to your success[9]. Studies have shown that a well designed diet can greatly improve your body's ability to adapt to strength training and increase muscle mass[156]. Starting with our energy equation (energy in must be greater than energy out), you must consume more calories than you burn per day. Start by adding 200 to 1000 calories a day to your diet[5, 9, 52, 71]. This can be achieved by adding meals, increasing the portion sizes at meals, or adding more snacks to your diet[9, 30, 52, 71].

Note: More than 1000 extra calories per day will likely increase your body fat. You can only construct a finite amount of muscle tissue per day[52]. Genetic potential, your exercise program, the amount of rest and recovery allowed during your program, and the degree to which you increase your calories will have an effect on the speed at which you gain muscle tissue[5]. So be patient. Body builders often train for a decade or more before they attain enough muscle mass to be competitive. If you or someone you know continually loses weight or struggles to gain weight on a weight-gain program, it could be a sign of an underlying medical condition and you should consult a physician[71].

Myth #13: *More protein is better.*
What You Should Know: You can only use so much.

Protein should be 10 - 35% or your total diet[52]. Like all calories, excess protein will either be used as energy or stored as fat. It is likely that protein will make up the smallest percentage of calories in your diet.

Protein makes up the constituent parts of many structures, including bones, ligaments, hair, nails, teeth, muscles, and organs, and is continually used to build, maintain and repair these structures and body tissues. Proteins are used to make enzymes, hormones, and are essential to immune system function. They can also be used for energy when carbohydrates and fat do not provide adequate fuel.

Many have misconstrued protein's role in rebuilding muscle tissue to mean that the more protein you ingest the more muscle you will build. However, your body can only utilize so much protein, and will only construct a finite amount of new muscle tissue per day. Consuming more protein than required will not release previously untapped muscle building capacity[30]. Protein is the building block for lean muscle mass, but excessive amounts of protein will only result in increased fat storage.

The recommended daily allowance for protein is approximately 0.4 grams per pound of bodyweight. Research does support that athletes need more protein, but studies show that no more than 0.9 grams per pound will be useful for gaining muscle[9, 52]. You can assume a need between 0.4 and 0.9 grams per pound of bodyweight if you are currently working out.

So why do fitness magazines suggest 1-2 grams per pound of muscle mass? It's simple. They're biased. Most fitness magazines make a large percentage of their profit from the advertisement of supplementation. Protein powder manufacturers are going to make it seem like the only way to get enough protein is to use their product and a lot of it.

Interesting Tidbit: Carbohydrates are likely more important than protein for those who are trying to gain weight/muscle or increase athletic performance[71]. While you need protein to create muscle tissue, you also have to fuel the resistance training required to add more muscle mass. You want your body to utilize carbohydrates for this energy source not protein. In this way, an abundant source of carbohydrates spares your muscle mass, by preventing your body from utilizing protein for energy[52].

Are beans, peanut butter, and other nuts good sources of protein? Yes and no. Dietary protein consists of smaller parts known as amino acids. Eight of these proteins are termed "essential." They are deemed essential because your body cannot create them; you must get them from food sources. Some protein sources do not contain all of the

23

essential amino acids, making them "incomplete." Beef, poultry, fish, dairy, and soy products are "complete" protein sources by themselves. Generally, plant products other than soy are not. In order to attain all of the essential amino acids from plant products, one may need to eat a variety of foods or combine certain foods. Things like beans and peanut butter do contain a fair amount protein, but are missing certain amino acids. Peanut butter can be combined with whole grains (ex. a whole wheat bagel), and beans can be combined with rice to make them complete.

Note: Vegetarians who rely on plant sources for protein may need to research further into food combining, or possibly supplementation.

More on Myth #12: Healthy ways to increase your caloric intake [9,30,52,71]

Meals:

- Choose nutritious foods at meals such as pasta, rice, whole grain bread, fruit, vegetables, legumes, granola, sweet potatoes, lean meats and cereal with milk.
- Increase the frequency of meals.
- Increase the portion sizes of your meals or have seconds.
- Take advantage of your body's increased ability to absorb nutrients post-exercise by planning a meal within 90 minutes of your exercise routine[52]. This meal should likely be high in carbohydrates, as a significant reduction in glycogen stores has been noted post workout, and high carbohydrates meals have been shown to increase insulin and glucose concentrations over high fat meals[20].

Snack Ideas:

- Dairy products: yogurt, cottage cheese, glass of milk
- Fruit
- Peanut butter and whole wheat bread
- Juices
- Lunch meats (roll-ups and sandwiches)
- Tuna and crackers
- Smoothies with protein powder

Weight gainer and protein supplements may be helpful in acquiring the extra calories needed for weight gain. However, one should not exceed one supplement per day, as focus should be given to whole foods.

Fundamental Diet Principles:

- When speaking about diet and exercise we measure energy in calories. A calorie is a unit of energy. We consume calories through various sources of carbohydrates, fat, protein, and alcohol. (Carbohydrates, fats and proteins are collectively known as macronutrients.)
- Nutrition is the other half of a fundamental equation; **Energy In = Energy out.** All performance and weight loss goals must consider the amount of energy expended and the amount of energy consumed.
- All macronutrients are equally important. There is no macronutrient that is better than the others, or one that is our enemy. If you consume more calories than you need whether from protein, fat, or carb', they will be stored.
- We burn calories continually just to stay alive. Breathing, your heart rate, and digestion of the food you eat burns considerable calories. The amount of calories you burn increases as the intensity of your physical activity increases - you do not stop burning calories until you die.

- Body fat is essentially stored calories, you can think of body fat as an energy reserve. Every pound of body fat is approximately 3500 stored calories.
- Proper nutrition is essential to a healthy lifestyle. Optimal nutrition can improve your performance during physical activity and enhance recovery [5].

Chapter 2:
Hydration and Supplementation

Hydration plays a huge role in optimal performance. Heck, water plays a huge role in just keeping you alive. Water is approximately 60% of your total bodyweight, is vital for temperature regulation, and is essential in creating the environment in which all metabolic processes occur. Even a small amount of dehydration - say 1% of your bodyweight - can decrease athletic performance[4].

The Effects of Dehydration:

Water is a large part of our blood. Dehydration decreases blood volume, blood pressure and stroke volume (the amount of blood your heart pumps out with each beat). Your heart rate must increase to compensate. This in turn contributes to a higher rate of perceived exertion and less nutrients and oxygen reaching hard-working muscles. In short, your heart is working harder and getting less done. Some have termed the disproportionate decrease in stroke volume and increase in heart rate during activity "cardiovascular drift"[99, 127, 170]. Several studies have tested the effects of hydration as a means of preventing cardiovascular drift[99, 127]. It does not appear that ingestion of fluid during activity will prevent this change, but that proper hydration or euhydration (above normal levels of hydration) achieved *before* cardiovascular activity may help to reduce cardiovascular drift[99, 127, 170].

(Note: This by no means should deter any individual from ingesting fluids during exercise. Fluid ingestion during activity is important in preventing dehydration and heat related illness. However, there is little you can do to increase your performance during exercise if you do not ingest adequate amounts of water during your day.)

Dehydration also impairs your body's ability to transfer heat from contracting muscles to the skin's surface where heat can be dissipated to the environment[4]. This will cause a faster rise in core body temperature, which could lead to heat injury and add to one's perceived level of exertion.

Dehydration may disrupt electrolyte balance, decreasing muscular performance. And it could interfere with normal function of the nervous system[52]. For example, the electrolytes, potassium, chloride and magnesium are essential to muscle contraction and nerve conduction[9].

Where should we get water from?

1. Water itself is the easiest way to stay hydrated.
2. Foods, including fruits and vegetables.
3. Juices, coffee, tea, milk and even alcoholic beverages contribute to our hydration (note: they may also be a source of excess calories)[52].
4. Soda is a poor choice. Soda contains little if any nutritional value, and is full of empty calories. The carbonation in soda also tends to reduce the amount of fluid ingested.

Myth #13: *Bottled water is better than "tap."*
What You Should Know: Tap water is regulated by the EPA. Bottled water is not well regulated.

Bottled water is not inherently better than tap water. Many states do not regulate bottled water. But, tap water everywhere in the U.S. is regulated by the Environmental Protection Agency[52]. If you prefer the taste of bottled water and that will cause you to drink more, by all means drink bottled water. Bottled water will certainly cause weight loss around your "wallet line," but it may not be better for you.

Myth #14: *Coffee and tea dehydrate you.*
What You Should Know: Coffee and Tea do not dehydrate you.

Although coffee and tea may act as diuretics, the amount of dehydration caused by these beverages is not equivocal to the volume of the fluid. Caffeine has been shown to cause one milliliter of fluid loss per milligram of caffeine. Look at the math: 240 milliliter cup of coffee has 80 milligrams of caffeine, so there is still a net hydration of 160 milliliters[52]. Tea generally has half the caffeine that coffee has per volume. A man dying of thirst in the desert wouldn't turn away a cup of coffee, and there's no reason he should.

More on Hydration:

The primary objective for replacing fluid loss during exercise is to maintain normal hydration. One should consume adequate fluids during the 24-hour period before an event and drink about 500ml of fluid about two hours before exercise to promote adequate hydration and allow time for excretion of excess ingested fluid.

Chugging water is preferred to sipping as the fluid volume of the stomach has the greatest influence on gastric emptying[4]. That is, the more fluid you have in your stomach the faster it will be absorbed. During a workout a person should concentrate on drinking cool to warm water as it is ideal for fluid replacement. Also we typically drink insufficient volumes of water to offset sweat losses[4-5, 30, 99]. So drink more.

Complete restoration of a fluid deficit cannot occur without electrolyte replacement (primarily sodium) from food or beverage[4-5, 52]. This should probably occur in a meal before your workout as opposed to eating a bar or salty snack during your workout. The rate of gastric emptying is proportionately slowed with an increase in carbohydrate concentration above 8 percent[5].

During workouts lasting longer than an hour, you may want to consider drinking a sports drink during your workout[52]. Sports drinks are formulated to provide the body with carbohydrates and electrolytes lost during intense exercise. However, they do not provide enough carbohydrates to slow the gastric emptying discussed above.

How do you know if you're drinking enough water?

You can use urine color comparison to monitor your hydrations status. Your goal is to drink enough fluid so that your urine is clear to a pale yellow color. Bright yellow, amber, or green-tinged urine suggests dehydration[52].

Hydration Reccomendation[4-5, 52]:

- A minimum of 2.7 liters of water per day for women 19 years of age or older. (not including exercise recommendation)
- A minimum of 3.7 liters of water per day for men 19 years of age or older. (not including exercise recommendation)
- 500 ml of fluid should be consumed before exercise. (allows time for excretion)
- 150 to 350 ml of fluid should be consumed every 15 to 20 minutes during.
- Consume enough fluid to offset water loss during exercise. Approximately 16-24 ounces for every pound lost during exercise.

Myth #15: *Working out will help you get over your hangover.*
What You Should Know: The only thing that will get rid of your hangover is time, sleep, water and a nutritious meal.

Your hangover is caused, at least in part, by an overdose of a drug. It is going to take time for your body to produce enough of the enzyme responsible for the breakdown of alcohol, so that alcohol may be metabolized and excreted from your system. I have seen no evidence that suggests that working out increases the production of this enzyme.

Dehydration is a contributing factor to the dreaded hangover, and considering most individuals do not drink enough fluid during their workouts to offset sweat losses, it is likely that working out with a hangover will only increase your dehydration. This could make you feel worse after your workout. Not to mention, your work-out will likely lack the intensity and attention that is needed to take a step toward improving your level of fitness.

As well, ingestion of alcohol can exert a deleterious effect upon a wide variety of motor skills[173]. This could make working-out with a hang-over clumsy and dangerous.

Myth #16: *Alcohol and athletics go together like peas and carrots.*
What You Should Know: Alcohol and exercise mix like water and oil.

Alcohol exerts no beneficial influence on exercise[173]; however, some active populations have a higher drinking rate than there sedentary counterparts [61,112].

It seems to me that alcohol has three serious strikes against it.

- Decreased coordination and performance during exercise and sport.
- A source of empty calories, which can lead to weight gain.
- Increases your risk for various diseases.

Decreased performance

We have all experienced the drudgery of a trip to the gym or practice with a hangover. Generally you feel weaker, may not be able to lift as much weight, last as long on the treadmill, or find that you're uncoordinated, and clumsy. I do not know anyone who performs optimally with a hangover. Although all the causes of a hangover are unknown, we do know some of the contributing factors.

- Alcohol also acts as a diuretic. Alcohol may inhibit the release of the anti-diuretic hormones, ADH and/or Vasopressin. These hormones normally cause the kidneys to conserve fluids. The result is concentrated urine, leading to dehydration. Dehydration impairs almost every physiological function [4, 9, 30, 52, 173]. (See "Hydration" for more details)
- Do not forget that alcohol is a drug and part of a hangover is experiencing a mild reaction from an overdose of alcohol. It takes time for the body to metabolize and excrete the toxins in alcoholic beverages; usually longer than we would like. Some of these toxins are known as congeners. They can be found in varying amounts in different types of liquor, usually more so in darker liquors.
- Dehydration may also lead to electrolyte imbalance and decreased performance.
- Alcohol interferes with your brain's ability to perform routine functions, such as controlling sleep patterns. Generally, a contributing factor to a hangover is a lack of quality sleep.
- Alcohol can exert a deleterious effect upon a wide variety of motor skills, including an increase in reaction time, a decrease in hand-eye coordination, accuracy, balance, and complex motor coordination[173]. Many individuals take for granted the complex motor coordination and balance that is involved with a standard dumbbell press, a squat, walking on a treadmill, or catching a fly ball. With motor function impaired, you increase the chance of making a mistake, and a mistake in sports and exercise could lead to injury. Although on most occasions you have room for error, with slower reaction times, your body will be unable to compensate as effectively.

- Studies have shown alcohol to have an effect on resting glycogen stores[173]. This is likely caused by a decrease in liver function specific to glucose metabolism. This means a decrease in the fuel that is most important to exercise, and this reduction in blood glucose and the following hypoglycemia is going to contribute to the lethargic feeling of a hangover.
- Some studies have shown chronic alcohol consumption decreases androgen uptake into muscles post-exercise[152]. This androgen uptake is very important to muscle growth, and a reduction would likely decrease the gains normally attained through exercise.

Weight Gain:

Alcohol can be an abundant source of calories, which often leads to weight gain. Since alcoholic beverages provide little if any nutritional value it is truly a source of empty calories. With 7 calories per gram, alcohol has nearly as many calories per gram as fat (9 cal/gram). In a study done on 31 year old men and women alcohol was one of leading predictors of abdominal obesity[89]. Take a look at the graph below and try to calculate the amount of calories you ingested the last time you went out for a "couple" of drinks.

Drink	Caloric Content
Coors Light or Bud Light 12 fl oz	110 calories
Budweiser and Coor's "Extra Gold" 12 fl oz	150 calories
Whiskey Sour 6.8 fl oz	249 calories
Margarita 7 fl oz	280 calories
Martini 4.5 fl oz	279-378 calories (depending on proof of vodka)
Wine (Burgundy) 4 fl oz	92 calories
Wine (cabernet sauvignon) 4 fl oz	88 calories
Wine (Carlo Rossi white) 4 fl oz	80 calories

Increased Risk of Disease and Death

Chronic alcohol consumption has been linked to a multitude of health problems. Studies have shown an increase in resting and exercise blood pressure, provocation of heart arrhythmias, generalized skeletal myopathy, cardiomyopathy, pharyngeal and esophageal cancer, and brain damage[71]. In two separate studies chronic alcohol consumption was found to contribute to osteoporosis and fatigue fractures[61, 124]. Liver damage seems to be the most prominent disease related to alcohol abuse[9, 173].

Interesting Tidbits: The most frightening statistics on alcohol involve the sheer number of people who abuse alcohol in the United States. There is an estimated 10,000,000 adult problem drinkers with an additional 3.3 million in the 14-17 age range[173]. Alcohol is associated with more than half of all traffic fatalities and more than one third of all injuries[173].

Myth #17: *Everybody needs to supplement their diet with a vitamin or mineral supplement.*
What You Should Know: Most people need food, not pills.

Certain medical conditions, diet practices, and/or taste aversions can cause an individual to become deficient in a specific nutrient. Examples may include iron supplementation for women during pregnancy, protein supplementation for strict vegetarians, or calcium supplementation for the competitive athlete who does not like the taste of dairy products[52]. In any case, you should consult your physician and a registered dietician if you think you may have a nutrient deficiency. The rest of us just need to eat healthy food.

Myth #18: *Most supplements are effective, I should trust my local supplement dealer.*
What You Should Know: Writing this section of the book has changed my view of supplementation from skepticism to utter dismay. There is no doubt in my mind that the supplement

industry is a multi-billion dollar, bull-shit industry, with few exceptions!

So as a general rule, I steer far clear of supplementation. But, I seem to be the exception rather than the rule. Supplements are more popular than ever, and even high school athletes are hooked[50, 143].

What's Wrong with Supplementation

1. Because they are marketed as a food item they are not regulated by the Food and Drug Administration (FDA). That means no one is policing their effectiveness, purity, claims, or potential for risk.
2. There is a general lack of unbiased third party research to support any claims made by supplement manufacturers. Most "research studies" seen in magazines and advertisements are done by the company who manufacture the product and are inherently biased. Further, case studies, including the testimonials of individuals, represents the weakest form of research.
3. Those supplements that are effective are generally far too expensive for the small effect they have on your performance. (Ex. $700 - $1000 a year for a product that may increase your performance by less than 1 percent.) Personal training and education on program design strategies give you far more bang for your buck. HMB is a great example of a product that has some effectiveness, but in the amount that has been proven effective is way too expensive for the average consumer.
4. Most supplements are so new that long term studies are not possible. There are many supplements on the market that are so new that research has yet to be done, and long-term effects cannot be investigated. These products may hold the key to untapped levels of performance, or they may have terrible long-term side-effects. Supplementation must be weighed on the basis of risk versus reward. Unless you are performing at the highest levels of competition and rely on athletic

performance to pay your bills, it is hard to justify the risk and expense of supplementation, and at the highest level of competition many of these substances are banned anyway.

5. Many supplements have potentially harmful side effects when combined with other medications or certain food products. (example: ephedrine and beta blockers). The Anne Marie Capati vs. Crunch Gyms case is a tragic example. At 37 years old, Anne Marie Capati had a stroke during a training session. It is believed that a reaction between her hypertension medication and the supplement Thermadrine (containing ephedrine) is to blame.

6. Many manufacturers overstate claim, or generalize the effects of their product to include markets that will receive little benefit. An example of generalization: Gatorade is an extremely effective performance enhancer for intense endurance events lasting longer than an hour, and is effective as a recovery aid post exhausting intense exercise. Some of their advertising infers that Gatorade will enhance the performance of any activity, including pool, golf, and weight lifting. Although Gatorade is a great product, it will not enhance the performance of short duration events and lighter activity.

7. Supplements should be just that, supplements to a healthy diet. They should not be used to replace real food and good nutritional practices. If you eat garbage most of the time it is unlikely one drink, bar, or powder, is going to improve your performance. Improving your eating habits should precede any supplement considerations. A good diet is your foundation for better health, weight loss, and/or performance, supplements are minor details in comparison.

Two Dangerous Examples of Supplements: Anabolic Agents:

Anabolic agents are those agents that improve the body's ability to build tissue. Of course most individuals immediately relate the word anabolic to anabolic steroids, but many other substances can fall into this category. We all know steroids are very effective supplements, but we also know they pose severe health risks, are illegal, and are banned from most competitions. Growth hormone is a relatively new player in the hunt for bigger, faster, stronger muscles. Like steroids there is little doubt of their potential effectiveness, but they pose such severe health risk you would have to be insane to take them[18, 25, 106]. Some of the side effects include pathological enlargement of the internal organs, bone deformation, and increased risk of various cancers[52]. Like steroids, growth hormone is also illegal and banned from most competitions.

Pro-hormone Supplementation:

Pro-hormone, and hormone-releasing supplements, have been heavily marketed. Even Mark McGwire jumped on the "Andro" bandwagon for a time, of course, his admission to steroid and human growth hormone use have since overshadowed this. These supplements are supposed to be either a couple of biological steps from the real thing (steroids), or help the body to release more testosterone and other growth factors. This includes supplements like androstenedione (commonly referred to as andro), tribulis terrestris, DHEA, chrysin, L-cartinine, CLA, chondroitin sulfate, vandyl sulfate, and inosine. Although millions of dollars have been spent by athletes hoping for the next "creatine-like" supplement or a legal alternative to steroids, research thus far has shown these supplements to be ineffective at improving performance[22, 52, 54, 82, 87, 138, 161]. Some studies have shown that these supplements may even have very negative side-effects, such as testosterone to estrogen-conversion in male athletes, and an increased risk for cardiovascular disease[22, 82].

The Few Effective Exceptions:

Key Note: Supplementation of any product can only be deemed effective if it improves function when taken in quantities higher than what our diets provide.

- Vitamin, mineral, and or protein supplements prescribed by your doctor or nutritionist to alleviate a deficiency.
- A multi-vitamin for those who refuse to make better choices and eat a well-balanced diet. If you eat a well balanced diet a multi-vitamin is simply not necessary[5].
- Protein supplements (including whey, soy, glutamine, BCAA's) may improve recovery, but only if your diet does not supply you with enough protein. Whole foods are always preferred to supplementation[52].
- Sports Drinks and gels for endurance activity lasting an hour or more.
- Creatine monohydrate for strength training.

That's it. You can bag the rest of the items sold in your local vitamin store (Vitamin shops, GNC, etc.), and use them for landfill. Most products are nothing more than a modern day version of "snake oil".

Multi-Vitamins

Although there may be nothing wrong with a multi-vitamin/mineral supplement, they're simply not necessary. The American College of Sports Medicine's position on vitamin and mineral supplements is as follows: "Athletes will not need vitamin and mineral supplements if adequate energy to maintain body weight is consumed from a variety of foods[5]."

If athletes, with their rigorous training regimens, do not need a vitamin/mineral supplement, neither do the rest of us. The catch is many individuals refuse to eat a healthy well-balanced diet that includes a variety of foods, and poor eating habits can lead to nutrient deficiency. If you refuse to eat better, discuss taking a multi-vitamin/mineral supplement with your physician or registered dietician.

Vitamin E

Vitamin E has had a ton of press lately and rightfully so. Vitamin E along with vitamins A and C are known as anti-oxidants and protect us against free radicals.

What are free radicals? Free radicals are highly reactive byproducts of normal cellular metabolism. (Note: free radicals may also be taken into the body from outside sources). This highly reactive quality may cause damage to cells. This includes damage to muscle, connective tissue, skin, and because free radicals can damage cell membranes and genetic material they have been linked to the development of cancer.

Because of this "protection function," antioxidants, including vitamin E, have been sold as a supplement that may be "anti-aging," "a recovery aid," "flu and cold protection," or "cancer preventing."

Unfortunately research is inconclusive[8, 12, 52, 70, 114]. This does not mean we do not need vitamin E of course. It simply means that we do not need more than what a healthy diet already provides us.

Good sources of vitamin E include[52]:

- Flake cereals: Total, Special K, Product 19, Wheat Bran Flakes
- Nuts: sunflower seeds, almonds, hazelnuts, and peanuts
- Cooking oils: cottonseed oil, safflower oil, and corn oil

Exercise researchers have investigated vitamin E supplementation as a means of enhancing recovery, but studies have shown no decrease in muscle damage or an increase in performance with supplementation[8, 12, 24, 32, 133].

Other Vitamin and Mineral Supplements:

Although every vitamin and mineral is important and has its individual function, it is unlikely that you need more of any one vitamin or mineral; at least not more than a healthy diet can provide for you. Many vitamins and minerals have been touted as performance enhancers because of their individual function, but I could not find any research that suggested supplementation of a single vitamin or mineral would help you with your health/fitness goals. Studies on B-6, C, E, Iron, magnesium, and calcium supplementation were ineffective as ergogenic (performance enhancing) aids[38, 52-53, 131, 153, 166].

Protein Supplementation:

Due to false advertising, tricky wording, and the testimonials of chemically-enhanced bodybuilders, many individuals have the false perception that they need massive amounts of protein to improve their performance. Supplement manufacturers use these massive amounts to scare the consumer into thinking that supplementation is the only way to get enough protein. However, athletes generally get plenty of protein in their diets, and whole food sources are always preferred to supplementation[52]. Some individuals have circumstances that legitimize the need for protein supplementation, but they are the exception, not the rule. Examples include the vegetarian athlete, exercisers whose travel schedule makes it hard to eat right, and supplementing a meal due to taste aversions.

Various studies on protein supplementation have shown that supplementation increases branched chain amino acids (BCAA's) in the blood, creating a better environment for muscle growth. This may also increase time to exhaustion, and help to prevent a decrease in immune function during intense training[11, 31, 41, 72, 108, 137, 139]. However, none of these studies compared supplementation to ingestion of an equivalent amount of protein from whole food sources. Nor were athletes prescribed a diet that ensured adequate protein consumption before supplementation. Protein powder, amino acids, glutamine, BCAA's, etc., all provide your body with essential amino acids which are important to recovery from exercise. However as discussed previously, your body can only utilize so much protein at a time.

The cost of protein powders and bars should also be considered. Whole foods are generally cheaper per gram and provide you with other essential nutrients. Compare the cost of chicken at 7 grams of protein per ounce, with a designer protein powder that may cost twice as much per gram. Supplement manufacturers will often try to fool the consumer into thinking quantities are larger than they really are by listing protein per serving in milligrams (1000mg = 1gram).

The recommended daily allowance for protein is approximately 0.4 grams of protein per pound of bodyweight. Research suggests that no more than 0.9 grams per pound will be useful for gaining muscle[9, 52]. As a recreational athlete or exerciser you can assume a need between 0.4 and 0.9 grams per pound of bodyweight.

> **Myth #19:** Sports drinks will enhance any activity.
> **What You Should Know:** Using drinks, bars, and other carbohydrate supplementation has no effect on activity lasting less than 1 hour [100, 118, 129].

Intermittent and shorter duration activities do not deplete the body enough to make these supplements necessary. Ingesting these supplements when unnecessary only adds calories to your diet and may contribute to weight gain.

Carbohydrates, Electrolytes and Water:

The popularity of marathons, cycling, triathlons, and field sports has created a market for products that enhance our endurance performance. Most supplements are unnecessary and ineffective; a few are potentially harmful, but there is a small group of supplements that has made getting essential nutrients more convenient.

Your body relies on sugar to fuel high intensity endurance activities, and water and electrolytes lost in sweat are essential to function. Carbohydrates, electrolytes (sodium, potassium, calcium, magnesium) and water could be consumed during activity with soy milk, bananas, and salt, but salted bananas in soy milk may be less than appetizing during a long, hot workout. Sports drinks, gels, bars and powders, are convenient ways of packaging these nutrients so they are easy to consume during activity.

Studies show carbohydrate ingestion during endurance activities lasting more than an hour, significantly improves performance, and sports drinks (w/ added electrolytes) can even improve physical and mental skills during the late stages of sports like basketball, tennis, and soccer [5, 42, 151, 167].

Tips for Optimal Use:

Sports drinks are likely a better choice than bars, powders and gels. The rate your stomach empties fluids into your body is slowed with an increase in carbohydrate concentration above 8 percent[5]. Sports drinks contain less than 8% carbohydrate, whereas, bars, gels, and powders are concentrated carbs, and require that you drink a significant amount of fluid to ensure that your stomach empties as quickly. Studies show that ingestion of carbohydrate drinks in the first hour of exercise improves time till exhaustion, so start drinking at the beginning of your workout[146]. Don't forget to look at the label and find sports drinks that use a variety of sugars (ex. glucose, fructose, and sucrose). This will improve your endurance performance, and make it less likely that consuming a large amount will cause nausea[80].

Recovery:

Knowing that sugar (carbohydrates) plays such a significant role in fueling our workouts it should be no surprise that carbohydrate ingestion post work-out is important to recovery. Carbohydrate post-workout is instrumental in restoring sugar stores that are utilized during workouts, and will improve cardiovascular performance in subsequent workouts. Note: There is likely no difference between a single meal and several smaller meals[119, 135].

Fat and protein cannot replace the carbohydrate.

Because fat is our largest energy reserve, and fat in food is calorically dense, many studies have examined if a diet high in fat will increase endurance performance. Although most studies show no decrease in performance, most show no increase in performance either[26, 28, 65, 68, 117, 141, 155]. I could only find one study that compared endurance performance on a high protein diet. The short-term diet plan did not decrease performance; however, no increase in performance was attained either[164]. Studies on diets that contain as much as 53% fat show little effect on endurance performance, providing they supply ample carbohydrates[23, 92, 155]. It is likely that the body can adequately adapt to a variety of macronutrient profiles, provided your diet supplies you with a minimum amount of carbs, fats and proteins. Ketogenic or low-carb diets would be examples where the macronutrient profile is so unbalanced that your performance is likely to suffer. Studies have shown that low-carb diets may allow you to maintain your current level of cardiovascular fitness, but it is unlikely you will be able to increase your performance[67, 68].

Other Supplements:

Most of the research I found on supplementation for cardiovascular performance tested stimulants. The stimulants in these studies included - caffeine, lepidium, meyenni, synephrine, jeevani, guarana, panax notoginseng (ginseng for short), mahaung, and ephedrine. Many of these substances are the active ingredients in various diet pills, such as Ripped Fuel and Trim Spa, or energy drinks like Red Bull, and Agent Orange. In a word; ineffective. Studies noted an increase in heart rate and blood pressure during endurance exercise which could potentially decrease endurance, increase your level of perceived exertion, and increase cardiovascular risk[39, 97, 102]. The supplement creatine has traditionally been used to enhance strength training because it aids our short-term energy systems. But, it has also been tested for cardiovascular activities. So far studies revealed that creatine has no effect on cardiovascular performance, even when periods of high intensity sprinting were added to a long distance run[16, 139].

> **Myth #20:** *Creatine will enhance your performance.*
> **What You Should Know:** Creatine alone will not improve a single lift, set, sprint, or power movement[6, 37, 60, 69, 116].

Creatine monohydrate is the supplement that everyone in the athletic community had been waiting for. It is considered a true performance enhancing agent. And the best part; unlike steroids, EPO, or growth hormone, there appears to be very little risk of side-effects. The continued popularity of creatine (nearly two decades) has led to an abundance of third party, unbiased research and an objective understanding of creatine's effects. Although exaggerated claims by supplement manufacturers deserve scrutiny, this is one of the few supplements that I can endorse.

Supplementing a diet with creatine monohydrate increases stored creatine phosphate within muscle tissue. Creatine phosphate is an energy molecule essential to short intense bouts of muscular exertion. A set of heavy bench presses is an example of this type of activity. The increase in stored creatine phosphate allows an individual to do a couple more reps before feeling fatigued. This leads to an increase in total work output during training[1, 33, 81, 83, 86, 94, 125, 162], and is especially effective at reducing decay and increasing performance during repeated sets of exercise, such as seen during training[33, 83, 86, 162]. This is not to say that you will be able to lift more weight, per se, you will simply get a small increase in the total reps you can perform with each set. It is likely that the increase in work output (load, volume, reps till failure, and decrease in decay with repeated sets) during training is the cause of mass, muscle, and performance increases seen with creatine supplementation[6, 123, 158].

Still creatine monohydrate is not magic. The value of creatine is realized when used as a workout or training enhancer. Any gains in performance are generally noted many weeks after beginning creatine supplementation and can be attributed to the increases in work output during training supplemented with creatine use; this is supported further by the relative ineffectiveness of short term use (6 days or less)[46, 59-60, 69, 93, 109, 116, 121]. This in no way under values the effectiveness of creatine monohydrate as attenuated strength gains during resistance training have been noted in several studies[13, 21, 29, 81, 83, 86, 158, 174]

Interesting Tidbits: Creatine has no effect on muscle and strength gains during highly structured resistance training programs (ex. college sports programs) where load, reps, and total volume are preset[51, 144, 169]. If you intend to use creatine you must perform activity until voluntary failure, and increase your volume (load and reps) over time. Also creatine has little to no effect in highly trained competitive athletes[37, 63, 110, 162]. This may be attributable to the "peak" performance that competitive athletes reach; similar to handing a climber a better pair of snow boots at the top of Mount Everest.

Myth #21: *You need 20g of creatine per day your first week and 6g every day after.*
What You Should Know: 3 grams a day is just as effective.

A loading phase of 20 grams per day is simply unnecessary; 3 grams has been shown to increase creatine stores to similar levels given time[6]. Even using 6-8 grams of creatine per day resulted in almost half being excreted in urine[27]. Interestingly, this study used a sample of division 1 college athletes during off-season training. These elite athletes do their highest volume of resistance training in the off-season which would seem to support a fairly large dose, but that was not the case. Evidently, we are limited in our ability to utilize this supplement. We can likely blame greedy supplement manufacturers and biased research for exaggerated doses.

Interesting Tidbit: Studies have also shown that creatine storage remained elevated for a month after supplementation stopped[122, 159].

Myth #22: *Creatine will lead to dehydration, cramps, renal problems, and other side effects.*
What You Should Know: Creatine is safe.

The only consistent side effect of creatine use is weight gain, specifically fat free mass[6, 21, 81, 83, 86,88, 94, 104,158-159, 174]. This could be detrimental to certain athletes, but it is hardly dangerous. For example, creatine does not improve swim performance[36, 109]; as added weight creates an increase in drag and reduces buoyancy.
Debunking other claims:

- There has been no evidence of dehydration or cramping with creatine use[6, 154].
- There seems to be no effect on renal function (even with 5 years of use) [104, 121].
- Creatine has no effect on blood pressure, plasma CK, hormone levels, cortisol levels, and does not seem to cause gastrointestinal problems[6, 47, 104, 157].

Resistance training and the effectiveness of sports drinks, energy bars, gels, and powders:

Carbohydrate supplements, such as sports drinks, do little to improve resistance training performance even when training lasts as long as 2 hours[149]. The two plausible exceptions to this rule are:

- Training sessions that use very high rep schemes with little to no rest between sets[62].
- Individuals who do multiple bouts of resistance training a day may improve recovery by ingesting a sports drink during resistance training[64].

A Note of Caution: Motivation and Behavior.

People engage in various dieting practices for a multitude of reasons. Various social stressors, psychological factors, economic situations, integral traits, level of physical activity, and the habits developed in an individual's youth may all have an impact on an individual's success at attaining their goals and their mental health during dieting[10, 34, 71, 77, 147, 168]. Social stigma, athletic performance, health, and/or vanity may all be motivating factors behind a weight-loss strategy, and careful consideration must be given to what drives an individual. It is important to understand that every individual is different.

Not all motivating factors for weight loss are positive. Our obsession with it does have costs and consequences. Some individuals are undergoing dangerous surgeries, adopting destructive eating disorders, over-exercising, incurring serious financial expense, and/or are suffering from psychological consequences[98]. The media has been no help in this arena. The average sizes of a playboy centerfold decreased significantly from 1958 to 1979, and although the trend did not continue into the 1980's, most models were of a low body weight. During that same decade, miss America contestants continued to get thinner, with nearly 69% of the contestants were15 percent below the normal weight for their heights[98]. Similar trends have been noted in a variety of magazines including <u>Seventeen</u> magazine, marketed as teenage girl's best friend[98]. More and more articles have appeared in magazines about diet and exercise emphasizing that dieting will improve appearance and increase attractiveness. Special care must be taken so that a healthy lifestyle change does not turn into a dangerous obsession. In two reviews on weight loss strategies and health and longevity, it was noted that lifestyle change was more important than weight loss[56, 105].

Care must be taken to refrain from negative feedback. That includes self-deprecating comments as well as negative and nagging statements given to or received by others. Negative stimulus from a loved one may turn healthy motivation to lose weight into a devastating obsession or an eating disorder. Even elite athletes may succumb to the pressures parents, coaches, and competition can put on them and adopt destructive disordered eating patterns. This is often seen in athletes involved in figure sports, and sports with weight classes[9, 154]. Just long-term dieting itself may have an effect on mood and psychological well being as seen in a study on female bodybuilders on restrictive diets[113].

In one study, it was noted that lower income individuals were more likely to be overweight and participate in sedentary leisure activities[34]. Although often attributed to "laziness," a lack of resources may make it hard to afford a gym membership, make education on fitness hard to acquire, and may make a healthy diet a financial burden.

The treatment of obesity must be addressed by professionals of various disciplines. Research indicates, nutrition, exercise, and consultation with a mental healthcare professional will all be important steps in recovering from obesity. This is not often a short-term battle as many studies show an increased rate of success with long-term intervention and follow-up[3]. Unfortunately, studies have shown that obese individuals are far less active than their healthy weight counterparts[171]. A general improvement in self-esteem, self-efficacy, and various health parameters is noted when obese individuals make positive lifestyle changes[71, 140]. Targeting behavioral processes and physical activity self-efficacy during intervention has resulted in increased success for weight loss in overweight women[57]. Intrinsic motivational factors, such as enjoyment and interest in exercise have been correlated with a successful weight loss strategy[145].

In today's remote control society, our environment has become conducive to less activity than previous generations. Greater food availability and "super-sized portions" have increased our overall caloric consumption[3]. We have to do our best to limit these factors and battle back against them. I know the method I put before you is not the easiest, and it is probably not anywhere close to what you wanted to hear, but it is the truth. Lifestyle modifications in food and exercise remain the hallmark of effective weight loss[71].

SECTION II:
THE TRUTH BEHIND
GETTING PHYSICAL

Chapter 3:
Spot Reduction

Myth #23: *You can target your fat parts.*
What You Should Know: You cannot target fat.

Where can you expect to lose fat? Everywhere and nowhere specifically. Studies show weight loss reduces fat stored in *all* parts of your body[32]. Although you may lose more fat in some areas, and less in others, it is currently believed that the *pattern* of fat loss is genetically predetermined[71]. If you have ever lost a significant amount of weight you may have noticed that your ring, shirt collar, and watch size changed along with your pant size.

Research has tried to determine a pattern to body fat loss, but results have been relatively inconclusive. Some studies have shown that *exercise* induced weight loss preferentially decreases abdominal fat over diet alone, but beyond this trend little has been determined[23, 30, 49].

Further, some fat is more than skin deep. One study showed that more visceral fat (the fat around your organs) was lost than subcutaneous fat (the fat just under the skin and over your muscles) during an eight week exercise program[17]. This may result in a smaller waist line without a significant impact on muscle definition. Although this may sound discouraging, be patient. Your body will continue to use fat from all parts of your body and contribute to a more defined appearance all over.

Myth #24: *Products that target my inner thighs, abs, and back of my arms are an important part of my exercise routine.*
What You Should Know: Don't waste your time.

"Toning" exercises may be effective for strengthening the muscles in your trouble spots, but they will not target the fat that covers them. Spot-reducing exercises like crunches, leg lifts, leg curls, and triceps extensions rely primarily on sugar to fuel activity, not fat. In fact, all resistance training (i.e. weight lifting) is fueled by sugar. The calories burned during these activities will have an impact on your total fat loss; however, small muscles burn fewer calories.

Exercise Tip: Stick to large movements

Many "toning" and "shaping" programs focus on the little muscles, but little muscles burn little calories. If we stick to large movements such as leg press, push-ups and rows we can maximize the amount of muscle utilized ensuring that more calories are burned and more muscle is added. Many of the small muscles that are targeted in shaping routines are naturally used during larger movements.
For example:

- Your inner thighs, outer thighs, and butt are extremely important to proper mechanics during a leg press, squat, step-up or lunge. There is no need to disassemble these movements into individual muscles. If you do one of the movements listed, you have worked all of the muscles in your legs and burned more calories in the process. If you want more work to do, pick two of the movements.
- Many individuals spend time working their arm muscles. However, your arms are included during pushing and pulling. For example a chest press not only works your chest, but it also works the front of your shoulders and the back of your arms as well. A seated-row works your entire back, the back or your shoulders, and your biceps.

- More advanced exercisers may add "integrated exercises" to their routine. Integrated exercises are a combination of upper and lower body exercises put together in a functional pattern. Examples may include a squat-to-row, step-up-to-curl-to-overhead press, or lunge to chest press. These exercises are very challenging, use a lot of muscles, and burn a tremendous amount of calories.

Why is it that women store more fat in their hips and thighs, and men store more in their mid-section?

In the hips and thighs of women, enzyme activity that initiates fat storage is very high and the enzyme activity for the breakdown of fat is relatively low. However, in the last trimester of pregnancy and throughout lactation, this enzyme activity changes increasing fat utilization in the hips and thighs. This suggests that this trend in fat storage may be important for reproductive purposes[11].

Although I could not find specific research concerning fat storage in men, I would assume that the enzyme activity responsible for fat storage in the midsection of men is similar to the hips and thighs of women. This would ensure that fat is deposited close to one's center of mass. Excess weight stored closer to your center of mass has less impact on daily movement. In a study examining weight distribution, an excess load on the foot changed walking mechanics and increased metabolism more than an identical load placed on the waist or thigh[50]. Example: If all of your fat was stored on your arms, how heavy would they be, how hard would it be to move them, and what impact would that have on your day? Even combing your hair could become a major chore.

How Does This Change My Workout?

Although you cannot target your trouble spots, you can be assured that a program focused on fat and weight loss will help you reduce body fat in all areas. You don't need to concern yourself with every little area and pick a specific exercise for each trouble spot. Keep your workouts fun, intense, and focused on the big picture. Try to maximize your caloric burn and focus on large movements that stress the major muscles of the body. Studies have shown that regular exercise increases your body's reliance on fat for fuel[43]. In other words, the more exercise you do, the better your body gets at burning fat. See "Some Pointers for Maximum Definition" in the next chapter for exercise tips guaranteed to burn more calories.

Chapter 4:
Toning

Myth #25: *Tone up those flabby muscles.*
What You Should Know: Tone does not mean what you think it does.

Everywhere I turn, I find myself surrounded by magazines, videos, and various devices that will tone-up my flabby midsection, my drooping butt, or flapping arms. "Tone" is not a myth, however when used in this context the word has been misinterpreted. Thanks to the popular media, misinterpretation of this word has led to misinformation and ineffective exercise suggestions.

I believe the misinterpretation stems from the belief that muscle tone and muscle definition are one in the same. This is not the case. Muscle definition is an adjective describing how good a muscle looks. Muscle tone is a word describing an aspect of neuromuscular motor behavior. All properly functioning muscles have an inherit amount of tone or tonus.

What is tone?

- **Tone** - The normal degree of vigor and tension; in muscle, the resistance to passive elongation or stretch; tonus.

- **Tonus** - The *slight, continuous contraction of muscle*, which in skeletal muscles aids in the maintenance of posture and in the return of blood to the heart. The normal condition of tension in muscles, making possible response to a stimulus.

Definitions from Dorland's
Illustrated Medical Dictionary.

This slight continuous contraction is vital for our working muscles. This is how muscles maintain our posture against the force of gravity and how they stay ready to contract. They need to be in constant preparation to contract so that we may respond to our environment in a timely manner and move efficiently. It's like keeping your car motor running while you're stopped at a red light. You wouldn't shut off the motor. If you did, you couldn't respond to the green light in a timely manner.

Increasing your muscle tone so that your muscles appear "more contracted" or an increase in muscle tone to increase your response time is not a feasible goal. Muscles must maintain balance with each other. An increase in the tone of one muscle often means the reduction of muscle tone in another. In fact, increased muscle tone is often a sign of injury, muscular imbalance, and movement dysfunction[10, 12].

Muscles can be over-active or under-active, that is have too much tone or too little.

- **Hypertonia** - A condition of excessive tone of the skeletal muscles; increased resistance of muscle to passive stretching. Hypertonic exhibiting hypertonia

- **Hypotonia** – A condition of diminished tone of the skeletal muscles; diminished resistance of muscles to passive stretching. Hypotonic: exhibiting hypotonia.

Definitions from Dorland's Illustrated Medical Dictionary.

An example of hypertonia:

After shoulder surgery, I started feeling a radiating pain from the base of my skull to the top, inside corner of my shoulder blade. My neck had become stiff and often cracked and popped when I turned my head from side to side. I saw a physical therapist who noted that the muscles that go from the base of my skull to my shoulder blade had become *hypertonic or overactive*. This is a common after shoulder injury, as these muscles are essential in maintaining the normal mechanics of your shoulder girdle. This does not mean that I had "ripped" traps and neck muscles, or that these muscles had become more visible. What it did mean was that these muscles had become overactive and would not shut off. This continuous contraction was overworking these muscles and they were becoming irritated and sore.

Will the exercises I see in fitness magazines improve my muscle tone?

No. I have found no research that suggests that resistance training alone will increase muscle tone.

Can I look more "toned"?

Yes, of course, but let's replace the word "tone" with "muscle definition".

How do I define my body?

Decrease your body fat and increase your muscle mass. Be more active, stick to a healthy diet, and begin a resistance training program to increase muscle size.

Can I work specifically on defining my abs or target my inner thighs?

No, this is commonly referred to as "spot reduction" or "spot toning", and unfortunately reducing your body fat in only one area is not possible. See "Spot Reduction" in the previous chapter.

Working muscles in one area may increase the size of those muscles targeted, but that hard work will not show until you reduce your body fat.

Myth #26: *More reps and lighter weights make you more defined.*
What You Should Know: More reps and lighter weights will not affect your appearance unless you do more total work.

More repetitions per set does not increase your muscle tone, but if more repetitions leads to more total work (reps x sets x weight), you will burn more calories. More calories burned means fewer calories stored. Fewer calories stored means less body fat. And, less body fat will give you a more defined appearance.

More on muscle tone?

Is there anything else you can do to improve your muscle tone? Yes, but it's complicated. Research suggests that postural distortion and injury may decrease muscle tone and lead to a decrease in muscle function[10, 12, 46]. This decrease in function could lead to a decrease in muscle size and affect appearance.

Getting a little deeper:

Muscle tone may be influenced by poor posture, injury, level of muscular fatigue, training status of the individual, the relative stability of the environment, specific forms of resistance training, and various forms of flexibility training[4-5, 10, 14, 16, 24, 27, 29, 33, 46].

Your health/fitness professional may utilize these variables to improve your posture, alter muscular recruitment patterns, and improve function, with a well designed program. These techniques and variables can create an optimal level of performance in all your working muscles, and therefore, an optimal amount of tone. To truly take advantage of these training methods that increase or decrease your muscular tonicity, you will need to enlist the help of a qualified fitness professional.

Injury:

For problems stemming from injury, it is important to follow a progression of treatment starting with an orthopedic physician, followed by physical therapy, and finally work with a qualified fitness professional to modify your existing workout plan. In a study examining individuals with ACL deficiencies there was an alteration to quadriceps (thigh muscle) recruitment, and the possible loss of tonicity even years post treatment[46]. In this study, an injury to the knee affected thigh muscle tone even years after the injury. Other injuries may create similar problems in various regions of the body and require the help of qualified professionals.

Postural distortion:

Postural distortions are very common and often arise from the tasks of daily living. For example, sitting at a desk all day, wearing high heels, or sleeping in the fetal position may cause tightness and joint dysfunction in the lower body. Joint dysfunction may lead to a decrease in muscular tone and affect appearance. Try standing and sitting with better posture, take off any shoe with a heel, and incorporate a flexibility program into your existing routine. If you enlist the help of a fitness professional and think your posture could use improvement, list "improve posture" as a priority when discussing your goals.

High Rep Training for Maximal Caloric Burn:

Often termed "muscular endurance" training, workouts that focus on higher repetitions increase your body's ability to sustain a muscular contraction. When training for better definition, these workouts have an added benefit. The high volume (reps x sets x weight) burns more calories than other forms of resistance training. Higher reps will not "tone" you up, but a high volume workout may burn more calories. To benefit from strength/endurance training we must pay attention to detail.

The keys to successful strength endurance training:
1. Time under tension:
   - Select a weight that allows you to perform 12-25 repetitions at a slow controlled tempo. Your muscle should be under continuous tension for 60 to 120 seconds. Note: They key word is *time*. 20 reps at a fast tempo and 10 reps at a moderate tempo may work the muscle for a similar amount of

time. We want to increase the amount of time our muscles are under stress increasing the calories we burn.

2. Lighter weight does not mean feather weights:
   - The weight utilized must create momentary muscular fatigue in 25 reps or less. If the weight is appropriate, you should not be able to do a 26th repetition. The body must be challenged to force change.

3. Less rest between sets.
   - The suggested rest period for endurance training is 30-60 seconds between sets[10]. We need to keep moving to continually burn calories. A stopwatch can be a wonderful tool in the gym, and may help you take your workouts to the next level.

Suggested parameters for endurance: guidelines set forth by the American College of Sports Medicine, the National Strength and Conditioning Association, and the National Academy of Sports Medicine[2, 10, 22].

Goal: Muscular Endurance/Fat Loss
Number of Exercises: 8-10 focusing on all major muscle groups
Sets: 1-3
Reps: 12-25
Rest: 30-60 seconds
Tempo: Slow (2 seconds up, 2 second hold, 2 seconds down)

Circuit Training:

Circuit training is a great way to set up a strength/endurance routine. A "circuit" is simply three or more exercises done back to back without rest. In essence you perform an exercise for a different muscle while the muscle you just worked is resting. It is a very efficient way to train, working more muscles, and burning more calories in less time.

For example you may choose an exercise for:
1. Legs
2. Chest
3. Back
4. Shoulders
5. Core

Perform these exercises back to back without rest. Repeat up to three times as your fitness level improves.

Most commercial health clubs including New York Sports Clubs, 24 Hour Fitness, Bally's, and Equinox have a circuit of machines in their facility to make a full-body circuit training program easily accessible to all members.

An eight machine circuit following these guidelines may include the following:

- Leg Press
- Leg Extension
- Leg Curl
- Lat Pull Down
- Shoulder Press
- Chest Press
- Bicep Curl
- Triceps Extension

Remember, no rest between equipment, but repetitions should be performed in a slow controlled fashion.

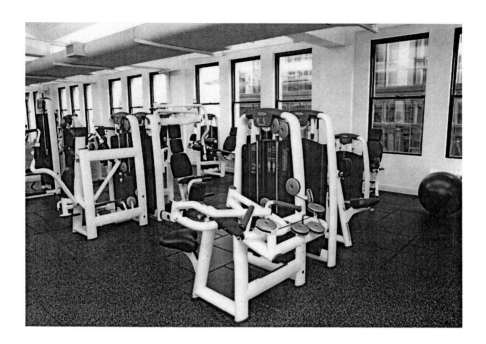

Choosing cardiovascular activity for maximum caloric burn:

When possible choose machines that keep you standing:
- Treadmills, elliptical trainers, and stair climbers generally burn more calories than bikes and swimming. The term "weight bearing" is utilized for exercise that is performed in a standing position. In essence, you have to move your entire bodyweight with each step. If your bodyweight is supported by a seat or the buoyancy of water you do not have to move as much weight and burn fewer calories.

If your arms are not moving than don't hold on:
- If the machine does not have moving arms, than try to maintain your balance without holding on to the machine. The increased work it takes to maintain your balance will burn more calories.

Try something new:
- If you keep doing the same thing, you'll keep looking the same way. Change may increase your caloric burn as your body works to adapt to the new exercise.

Try a class:
- Although it's not for everyone, many individuals get a better workout in a class setting. This is likely the result of peer-support or peer-pressure increasing your effort.

Competitive Sports:
- Many individuals are motivated to new levels of intensity in a competitive environment. Find a sport or activity you enjoy, a partner to enjoy it with, and have fun.

Chapter 5:
The Ab-solute Facts

Myth #27: *More abdominal work will get you a "six-pack."*
What You Should Know: You can't see through fat.

Everyone has a six-pack, the muscle is known as your rectus abdominis or "abs" for short. For most of us, it's hidden beneath a layer of fat. No matter how tight, "toned," strong, or big your ab muscles get, it's the fat that prevents most of us from seeing our six-pack. Training can increase the size and firmness of your abdominals, but you will not see a change in the appearance of your midsection. So remember, if your goal is to "tone up" or increase the muscle definition of your tummy, than the largest improvements will likely come with a reduction in body fat.

Abdominal Exercise:

1. Your abs and the muscles supporting your spine, often referred to as core muscles, are very important to your health and function. Exercise for these muscles should be incorporated into your resistance training routine.
2. In five separate studies comparing abdominal exercises, the crunch was found to stimulate your rectus abdominis more effectively than commercial devices.

3. In three separate studies, doing crunches on a stability ball created more muscle activity than the standard crunch. This is a great way to progress your abdominal exercise.
4. Your abdominal muscles do not attach to your legs - your abdominal muscles cannot raise, lower, or twist your legs in any way.
5. You cannot target your upper or lower abs. (Since you cannot spot reduce, i.e. target the fat on your lower abs, why would you want to?)
6. Commercial electric stimulators are not effective. They will not get you the abs you always wanted or shrink your waistline.

Myth #28: *Every fit person should have a tight, toned, six-pack.*
What You Should Know: Having a six-pack requires most people to maintain a body fat percentage well below a healthy norm.

Most of the individuals that I know who have six-packs do not have six-packs because they exercise with that specific goal in mind. They simply have incredibly active lifestyles that ensure body fat is burned like lighter fluid on an open flame. Those individuals who have six-packs have found a physical activity they enjoy and do it so often they have a harder time keeping weight on than taking it off. Think about it – basketball players, dancers, gym-rats, cyclists, and runners all relish in their daily physical activity. They literally have six packs by accident.

Somehow the "six-pack by accident athletic build" has influenced models, movie stars, and other media, and we are inundated with an unrealistic image of fitness. Having a six-pack has become the symbol of good health, but health and a visible rectus abdominis have very little to do with one another. The healthy body fat percentage for men is roughly 13-16 percent and women 20-25 percent[48]. I have never known an individual with a six-pack who had more than half the norm. How many individuals do you know personally, who have a clearly visible "six-pack?" I'm a fitness professional and I only know a handful. If a visible rectus abdominis requires you to cut your body fat to half of what is considered healthy, is it worth the work you will have to put in? I can't answer that question for you, but the question does force some serious thought about our goals.

At the end of the day, it is simply not necessary to be that lean. Fat does have a variety of important roles with in the human body, and excessive fat loss may lead to depression, interruption of the menstrual cycle, infertility, impaired temperature regulation, and even death[11]. Don't get me wrong, decreasing your body fat to normal levels is important. Studies show a link between abdominal girth and cardiovascular disease[12]. However, there is a strong distinction between a smaller healthier waist line and a six-pack.

A note of caution:

Our vanity may be what condemns us. Many individuals who I meet in the gym, I never see again. Many of these people are frustrated with their lack of progress or are overwhelmed by all the routines they have tried. Many of these routines promise results that are physiologically impossible. With every new routine that results in failure, motivation decreases. Eventually, many become bitter with the process and adopt a belief that the goal is not worth the price. Never forget that the real goal is health, not vanity. We are trying to add years to our lives and life to our years.

Myth #29: *You can work your lower abs.*
What You Should Know: There is no such thing as lower abs.

One of the largest myths in the fitness industry is whether or not you can target the upper or lower portion of your abs. Allow me to destroy this myth right now. All muscles contract from origin to insertion. That is your abs, when activated, will always contract across the whole length of the muscle from pelvis to rib cage. The muscle must contract across its full length to act on your spine effectively. You would never think of working your lower bicep or lower glutes, so why your lower abs? Imagine your abs are a rope that pulled your spine forward. Could you pull on one end of the rope without creating tension on the other end? Could you pull your spine forward before there was tension across the entire length? Could you pull on one end of the rope, and expect to accomplish anything if there was still slack in the line? Your abs work the same way.

Several studies comparing abdominal exercises and the activity of your upper and lower abs show that an increase in upper rectus abdominis activity does not occur without an increase in lower abdominal activity, regardless of the exercise[11, 38, 40-41, 45]. The two ends must work together. After all, they are the same muscle.

Getting far more technical. There are two nerve innervations for your rectus abdominis. Nerve innervations are like power chords; they transmit the signal from your brain that tells a muscle to "turn-on" or contract. One nerve intersects the lower rectus abdominis and one intersects the upper rectus abdominis. Put simply these two power chords seem to be plugged into the same switch. When either your upper or lower abs gets the "command" to fire, the other turns on as well.

There is a chance that the nerve to your upper abs and the nerve to your lower abs may be able to send separate levels of stimulation. Studies using electromyography, which records the electrical activity within a muscle, show the largest amount of activity during a concentric contraction – a contraction that causes a muscle to shorten against resistance. It takes slightly less stimulation to isometrically contract, or simply hold a position against resistance, and the least amount of stimulation to eccentrically contract, or let down slowly against resistance. With this in mind, if the upper abs just held tightly at the same length (isometric contraction) and the lower abs shortened against them (concentric contraction), we would have a gross shortening of your abdominal muscles and therefore movement. There would be a difference in stimulation between upper and lower portions of the rectus abdominis with a larger amount of stimulation in your lower abs. Keep in mind that both the upper and the lower abs are still active, there is just more "stimulus" in the lower abs.

The problem with this theory is application. In a single study, reverse crunches did create more stimulation in the lower abs than the upper abs. But the difference was not statistically significant, providing an inference to this phenomenon but not hard evidence[11]. I have yet to see another study comparing the activity in the upper and lower abs that gave concrete evidence that this phenomenon was possible. Although it may be great in theory, stay away from so called lower abdominal exercises such as lying leg lifts, hanging leg raises, and the roman chair leg raises. Generally these require your abs to hold a static length, and while you strengthen hip flexor muscles that may contribute to low back pain.

Myth #30: *When I do leg raises, bicycles, and flutter kicks I feel my lower abs.*
What You Should Know: You are actually feeling a muscle behind your lower abs called your psoas.

Many so called lower abdominal exercises involve leg lifts, bicycle kicks, or require you to bend at the hip (such as a sit-up). Your rectus abdominis muscle originates at your pubic crest (you can feel your pubic bone just above your "pubic area") and travels upward, attaching to the lower part of your ribs and breast bone. It does not attach to your legs or hips, so it cannot move your legs.

You may feel certain exercises in your lower abdominal region. Chances are, you are feeling a combination of your abdominal muscles and the deeper muscles of your midsection. During leg raises, knee ups, and bicycle kicks, the abdominal musculature must hold your pelvic bone steady. If your pelvic bone were to rock freely with your legs, your spine would have to bend vigorously and that could lead to low back pain and possible injury. Just as holding weight in front of you will make your shoulders burn, your abs burn as they attempt to hold your pelvic girdle steady during these leg movements. However, this still does not explain why the majority of sensation is in the lower part of your abs.

A powerful hip flexor known as your psoas lies just beneath your lower abdominal area and is responsible for lifting your legs. Your psoas is the prime mover (most responsible) for leg raises, knee ups, and bicycle kicks and this is likely the cause of the "burn in the lower abs." This is not an ideal way to increase strength in your midsection, and may be too effective for strengthening your hip flexors. Over development of your hip flexor musculature may reduce hip flex-ibility, causing posture problems and low back pain[22]. Because more than 80 percent of the population has or will experience low back pain[10], these exercises are not recommended for most individuals.

Myth #31: *You can shock your way to better abs.*
What You Should Know: Electronic stimulators don't work.

There are a number of devices on the market that use an electric current to work our abs while we sit behind a desk, watch TV or even sleep. I wish these devices worked. I would likely skip many a work-out in favor of "plugging in". Heck, maybe we could trade in hard work and exercise for licking a wall socket each morning. Before we open our wallets for one of these gadgets there are three problems to consider .

1. The level of electrical stimulation required to create growth or an increase in strength would be unbearably painful for most people, and a device that could deliver that level of stimula-tion would not be commercially available.
2. The amount of calories burned during this type of stimulation is unlikely to create a caloric deficit, which is what's necessary for the reduction in body fat that would make a six-pack visible.
3. There is no third party research that supports the use of com-mercially available electronic stimulators for this purpose.

The bottom line on this is pretty clean-cut: If it sounds too good to be true, it probably is. In one study, electric stimulation was found to be an effective means of increasing strength and size of the targeted muscle in novice exercisers[36]. But, the equipment they used was stronger than anything you could possibly purchase via infomercial. In fact, the current was so strong that candidates had to be tested for tolerance before the study could commence.

In a study using a common over the counter electrical muscle stimulation device (Bodyshapers model BM1012BI) subjects were tested for strength gains, body fat, girth measurements and were asked to assess their physical appearance over eight weeks. There was no significant change in any of the tested parameters[34].

Two other commercially available devices (Abtronic and Feminique) were also tested. The total caloric burn from using these devices would be approximately 36 calories a day if the device was worn 24 hours per day[19]. This is equal to about a half a slice of bread. If you wore this abdominal stimulator 24 hours a day, 7 days a week, it would take about three months to burn a pound of fat, and almost four years to burn off the freshman 15. (P.S. - That is not a suggestion.)

Myth #32: *Sweat away that belly fat with waist wraps.*
What You Should Know: Sweat isn't melted fat.

The excess weight you lose during this absurd method of training is water weight, not fat. The weight will return as soon as you ingest enough fluid to offset that lost during the activity. In a nutshell, you're losing weight, but the wrong kind, and it won't last.

The Core

Rather than creating a routine solely for your abs, you should concentrate on working all of your *core* muscles during a work-out. The *core* is the muscles of your midsection, spine, and hips, which are essential to stabilizing your spine, and transferring force between your upper and lower body. For many of us, it is also a symbol of health and beauty, but reducing your body fat, improving function, and increasing strength will take care of that.

Your core not only statically supports your hips and spine, but maintains alignment of your spine, pelvis, and hips during movement. All exercise and daily activity relies on your core to perform this function. Several studies have reported altered joint mechanics that could lead to injury when the core musculature does not perform optimally[1, 25, 28, 48].

Because a strong core will create a stable base and transfer the force you produce more efficiently, a strong core could be the missing link between how you perform now and a new level of performance. Studies have shown core strengthening may improve vertical jumping, gymnastics, your golf or baseball swing, as well as improving more general attributes of performance including balance, joint mechanics, and unilateral strength (activity that occurs on one leg, or pushing and pulling with one arm)[6, 8-9, 13, 21, 42, 47].

The previous chapter(s) may have left you a little confused as to which exercises will work best to strengthen your midsection, so let's rebuild your core program based on evidence and research to ensure you see change. We will focus on exercises that force you to stabilize your spine, flex your spine, extend your hips, and rotate your spine and hips. I chose the following exercises for their effectiveness in building core strength and addressing common weaknesses. I also chose exercises that for the most part, involve minimal equipment so that they may be done at home.

Plank:

A "plank" is a static stabilization exercise. It challenges your core musculatures ability to maintain alignment of the spine. A plank is performed in a face down position with the midsection elevated off the floor by your limbs. You must draw your belly button in and tighten your abs to maintain perfect alignment. You may want to arch up or let your back sway as your midsection is suspended, but you must maintain a neutral position. The challenge is to hold that position for 60 seconds or more without losing the drawing in maneuver, the tightness in your midsection, or your form. This exercise is named for the position resembling a stiff plank of wood. When progressing to straight leg variations: tuck your toes under you're your shins, draw in, tighten your abs, squeeze your glutes pushing through your feet and elevate your midsection until you are flat.

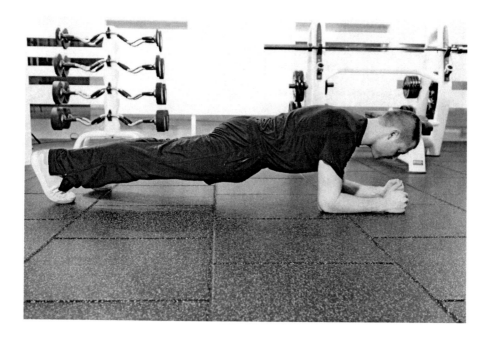

Crunch:

A crunch is a dynamic strengthening exercise for the muscles that flex your spine. This exercise is performed lying on your back with knees and hips bent so that your feet are flat on the floor, shoulder width apart, 6 to 12 inches from your butt. Your goal is to draw your belly button in and slide the bottom of your rib cage closer to your hip bones by slowly raising your shoulder blades off the floor. Your low back should not leave the floor during this exercise. Your hands can be placed in various positions to progress the exercises as you improve. For example: a crunch performed with hands on thighs is not as difficult as a crunch with hands outstretched behind you. Note: your abs do not connect to your neck, although your head will leave the floor you should always be facing the ceiling. Tucking your chin to your chest may put excessive strain on your neck.

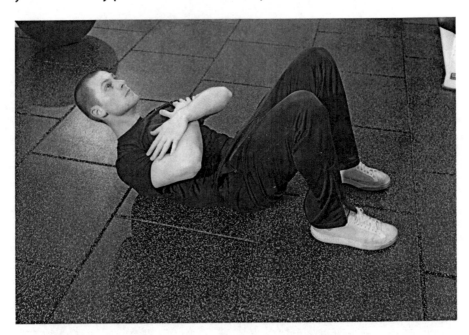

Oblique Crunch:

This is a dynamic strengthening exercise for the flexors and rotators of the spine. The technique is similar to a crunch, but with a twist. All of the same rules apply for this exercise. Rather than simply lifting your shoulders of the ground, you will twist by reaching towards the opposite knee with your hands, elbows or shoulder.

Bridge:

The bridge is a dynamic strengthening exercise for your butt muscles, and is a static stabilization exercise for the muscles of your low back. You perform this exercise while lying on your back in the same position as a crunch. Draw your belly button in, and squeeze your glutes, pressing your feet through the floor to lift up your hips. Lift your hips as high as you can without arching your low back. You should feel this exercise in your glutes. If you feel this exercise in your hamstrings restart the exercise with your feet closer to your butt. If you feel this exercise in your back restart the exercise, keeping your abs drawn in and contracted a little harder than your previous attempt.

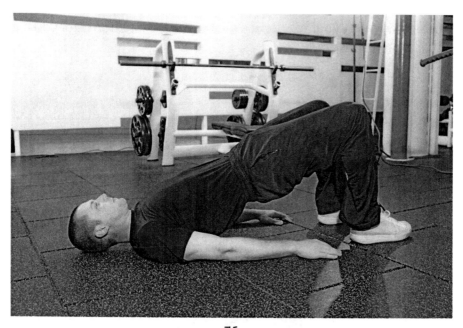

Adding the Stability Ball:

The stability ball is a great way to progress your core exercise. Your body must recruit more muscle fibers within your trunk musculature to stabilize your spine in an unstable environment. Studies have shown that exercise on a stability ball increases core muscle activation, increasing balance and strength[6, 11, 13]. But remember to pay attention to your form. Any exercise you are going to perform on a stability ball should be performed with optimal form on the floor or a bench before you progress. You can see examples of core exercises and progressions below.

Planks on a ball:

The technique used for planks on a ball is the same as the technique for the exercise done on the floor. But this time the ball will force your abdominals, hips, and shoulders to maintain alignment in an unstable environment. Center your forearms on the stability ball, push your elbows into the ball without allowing your chest to sag, draw your belly button in to tighten your abs, squeeze your glutes pushing through your feet, and elevate your midsection until you are flat as a plank of wood.

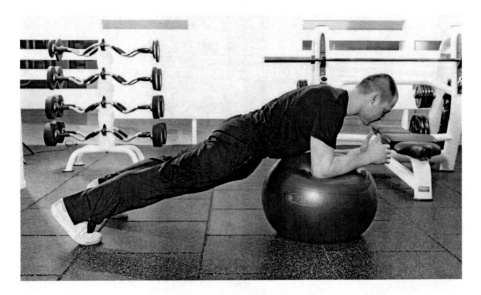

Crunches and Oblique Crunches on a Stability Ball:

Although the technique does not change, your position does. To acquire optimal results from this exercise, special attention needs to be given to form. You should find a stability ball that is knee high. Start by sitting on the ball and rolling down until your low back is centered on the ball. Adjust your feet so that they are shoulder width and directly under your knees. Lean back and squeeze your glutes to lift your hips up. Maintain a tight butt throughout the duration of the exercise. Keeping your hips high will ensure that you are focused on moving your spine forward and not your hips. Remember, spine movement = abs work, and hip movement = hip flexor work. The starting position should look like your best impression of a table, level, centered, with no warping. The exercise is then performed with the same techniques described above.

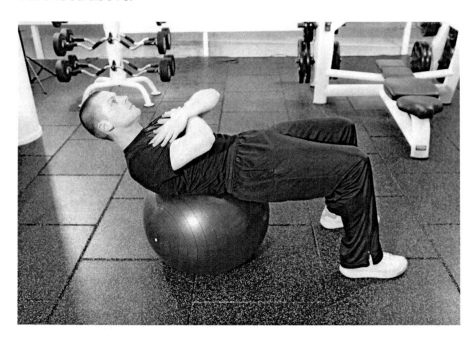

Bridges on a Ball:

Once again the technique utilized during this exercise is the same, however the position you are in differs. You should be able to perform floor bridges with perfect form before progressing to the ball. You should find a stability ball that is knee high. Start by sitting on the ball and rolling down until the ball is centered between your shoulder blades with your head resting in a neutral position on the back of the ball. Adjust your feet so that they are shoulder width and directly under your knees. Allow your hips to sink keeping your abs tight and back straight. Stop before you touch the floor. Squeeze your glutes pressing your feet through the floor and elevate your hips as high as you can without arching your back.

Prone stability ball cobra:

Lay face down over a stability ball with your feet against a wall. Center the ball on your hips and cross your arms across your chest. In the starting position you should have your feet flat against the wall, your knees bent but not touching the floor, your hips flexed allowing your thighs to rest against the ball and your chest curled over the ball. Draw your belly button to your spine and push yourself away from the wall. Squeeze your glutes pressing your hips into the ball and get as long as possible. The goal is not to get as high as you can off the ball, but to get long making your body as straight as possible, face down. Hold for a couple of seconds, slowly return to the starting position and repeat.

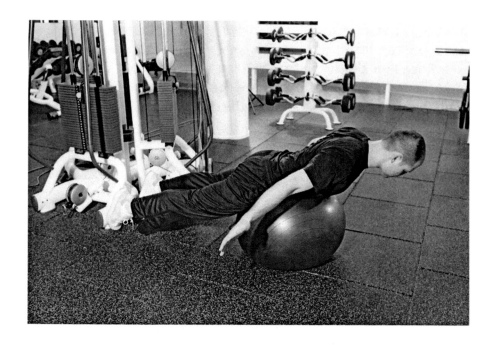

Advanced Movements:

Planks on ball with Knee Ups:

This exercise challenges your core musculature to statically stabilize your spine during leg movement. Center your hands on the sides of the stability ball, fingers pointing towards the floor. Get into a push-up position, by pressing your hands firmly into the ball not allowing your chest to sag. Draw your belly button in and tighten your abs, squeeze your glutes pushing through your feet and elevate your midsection until you are flat as a plank of wood. Bring your feet together so they touch one another and shift your weight to one leg by squeezing your tush and pressing that foot through the floor. Slowly elevate the opposite foot bringing your leg forward and touching your knee to the ball. Slowly return your foot to the floor and repeat on the other side. The challenge is to touch the ball with your knee and slowly switch from leg to leg without moving your trunk. You must maintain a tight midsection and perfect alignment of your spine and hips throughout the duration of the set.

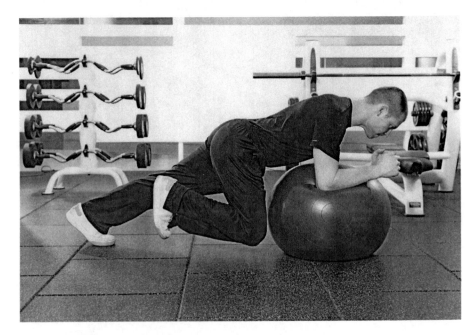

Resisted Crunch on Ball:

The position on the ball remains the same, and the technique is the same, however, the position of your arms will affect the difficulty of the exercise. You must be able to perform all variations of a crunch, both on the floor and on a ball before you attempt to add resistance to this exercise. You may hold a dumbbell or medicine ball over your chest with arms straight. The goal is not to raise the weight with your arms, but elevate the weight by crunching and lifting your shoulder blades away from the ball or floor. Remember gravity pushes straight down, so you should push the medicine ball or dumbbell straight up.

Rocking the weight back and forth as you crunch does not provide much resistance to the movement.

A more difficult variation would be to hold a light dumbbell or medicine ball in your hands with arms outstretched behind your head. Perform this variation maintaining your arms in line with your ears. Do not pull the weight over your chest as you crunch or the resistance created by your outstretched arms is lost.

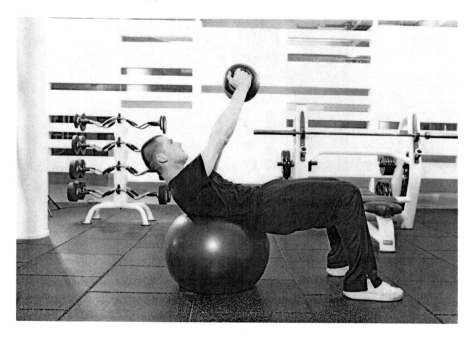

Single Leg Bridge:

The single leg bridge utilizes the same technique as the bridge on the floor, however you will keep one foot suspended a couple of inches from the floor and utilize the opposite leg to elevate your hips. This exercise requires much more strength from your glutes than the two-legged bridge. Special attention must be paid to lower body alignment. The hips must remain level and the leg that is being used to elevate the hips must stay perfectly aligned. You should be able to draw a straight line through your hip, knee, ankle and second toe.

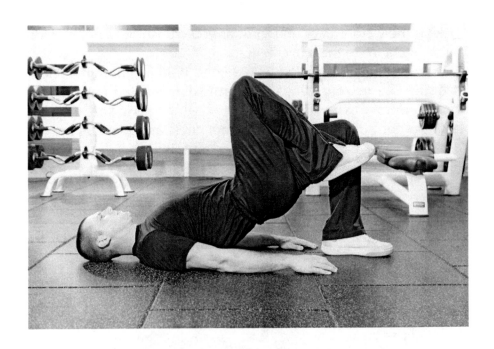

Axe chops:

Using a high cable column or an elastic band fixed to a high object, take a position facing perpendicular to the resistance. Take one small step back so the weight is now to one side and slightly in front of you. Stand up tall with feet shoulder width, pointing forward. Grab the handle of the band or cable with both hands and outstretched arms.

Assuming we start with the weight on your right side, allow the cable to pull your arms up and twist your shoulders to the right. In the starting position your hips feet and knees should remain in alignment pointing forward with rotation coming from your trunk and shoulders. Draw your belly button in, tighten your midsection, and bend and twist at the waist and hips as you pull the cable from in front of your shoulders down past your left hip. Your right foot should turn in creating a 90 degree angle with your fixed left foot at the end of the movement. Reach as though you were going to touch a point beyond your left toe. Slowly return to your starting position not allowing your feet and hips to go beyond the starting position. Repeat on the other side.

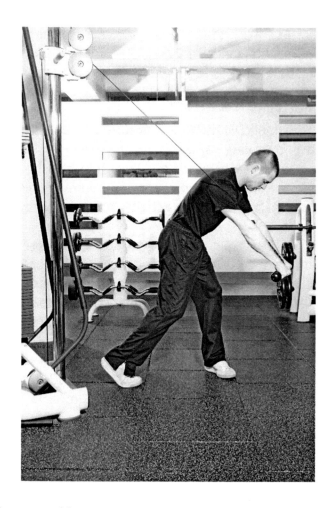

Myth #33: *Adding equipment to your ab exercises will get you better results.*
What You Should Know: Nothing beats the standard crunch for strengthening your six-pack muscle.

Why crunches are the best exercise for your six-pack muscle:

- The standard, bent knee, floor crunch stimulates the rectus abdominis as well as or better than the Ab-Doer Pro,

Perfect Abs, Perfect Abs Roller, Abs Roller Plus, Ab Sculptor, Ab-Trainer, Ab Works, Ab Scissor, Ab Swing, 6SecondAbs, Torso Track, Torso Track 2, leg lowering exercises, stability ball roll outs, reverse curl-ups, sit-ups, and crunches in which the feet were hooked[11, 15, 18, 40-41, 45].

- The crunch allows the rectus abdominis to contract through a more complete range of motion than rocking or pivot type devices – Ab Trainer, Abs Health Rider, Abs T45 and Ab Shaper[16]. A larger range of motion means more strength in all positions, more muscle activity, and possibly better results over time.

- Crunches are likely safer for those with lower back pain. Studies have reported those exercises that involve leg movement and those that lock the feet into position increase the activity of hip flexor musculature and decrease the activity of abdominal musculature[15, 18]. Over-development of hip flexor musculature could be a precursor to low back problems.

- The Ab-One was the only device that created a larger response during electromyography testing[40]. However, this device was designed to apply direct pressure to your abs as you do a crunch. That is, you crunch and push this hard piece of plastic into your stomach. If you manage to finish a set without throwing up or lacerating internal organs, you might make your abs sore. It could be bruising, but you'll be sore. It's thought to create a larger level of muscle activity as your abdominal wall increases tension to protect your internal organs, similar to how your abs tense if you get poked or punched in the belly.

Many of you have been doing crunches for years. So what's next? - *Progression* - Small progressions in difficulty add up to large changes over time. You must progress exercises to continue seeing results; however, before you can progress you must perfect!!!

"Practice doesn't make perfect, practice makes permanent. Perfect practice makes perfect."

1. Each exercise should be performed in a slow controlled fashion.
2. Draw your belly button in towards your spine at the beginning of each exercise and hold that "Drawing-In maneuver" throughout the duration of the exercise. Drawing in activates your deep core stabilization musculature.
3. Perform a minimum of 12 repetitions.
4. The exercise can be performed with perfect form through the whole set. No sloppy reps at the end to squeeze out a couple more repetitions.
5. If you can perform more than 25 repetitions you must progress to continue seeing results.

Building your core routine:

Once again, your core musculature can stabilize your spine, flex your spine, extend your hips, or rotate your spine and hips. If you choose an exercise for each function, perform those exercises in circuit, and progress on a bi-monthly basis (taking the time to perfect your technique), you could reach new personal bests. Note: you may not progress evenly through this graph. For example, you may find planks easy while needing more time to perfect your bridging technique.

As the weeks and months go by you may increase from 12 to 25 repetitions per exercise, and perform the circuit up to 3 times. But you should not increase the reps or sets if you cannot perform all repetitions with perfect form.

	Exercise 1	Exercise 2	Exercise 3	Exercise 4
Week	Stabilize	Flex	Extend	Rotate
1	Plank: On elbow and knees.	Crunch: Reach towards your knees.	Bridge: With hands on floor beside your butt.	Oblique Crunch: Reach one hand to opposite knee.
3	Plank On elbows, with one straight leg and one knee down.	Crunch: Arms folded across chest.	Bridges: Elbows down but bent so your hands rest on your belly.	Oblique Crunch: Arms across chest reaching elbow to opposite knee.
5	Plank: Only toes and forearms in contact with the floor.	Crunch: Fingertips behind ears with elbows back. Do not interlock your fingers behind your head. This may lead to pulling on the neck.	Bridges: Arms across chest.	Oblique Crunch: Crunch with a twist: Fingertips behind ears with elbows back. Crunch and twist as if trying to touch one shoulder to opposite knee.
7	Plank: Elbows and one foot. Raise the other leg only a couple of inches, pointing the leg straight back.	Crunch: Hands reaching behind you with elbows locked.	Bridges on ball: See description above.	Oblique Crunch: Hands reaching behind you, slowly bringing one arm forward to touch the opposite knee as you crunch.

9	Plank on ball: Up on your toes with forearms on ball.	Crunch on ball: Arms across chest.	Bridge on ball: With feet on a pillow or foam pad.	Oblique Crunch on ball: Arms across chest reaching elbow towards opposite knee.
11	Plank on ball: Hands on a stability ball in push-up position with one foot elevated 2 inches off the floor and pointing back. Switch feet.	Crunch on ball: Hands behind ears and elbows back.	Prone Cobra: See description above under "Adding a stability ball".	Oblique Crunch on ball: Fingertips behind ears aiming one shoulder to the opposite knee.
13	Plank on ball: Elbows on ball with one foot elevated inches off the floor and pointing back.	Crunch on ball: Arms reaching behind you with elbows locked.	Resisted Prone Cobra: Cobra holding a dumbbell or weight plate across your chest.	Oblique crunch on ball: Perform the crunch with arms behind you reaching one arm forward as you crunch to the opposite knee.
15	Plank on ball with hip hike: See description above, under "Advanced Movements".	Resisted Crunch on Ball: See description above, under "Advanced Movements".	Single Leg Bridge: See description above, under "Advanced Movements".	Axe Chop: See description above, under "Advanced Movements".

Myth #34: *For best results work your midsection every day.*
What You Should Know: Like all muscles, your midsection needs rest too.

Studies show that 2 – 3 times per week is effective for strengthening our core musculature[51-52]. Forty-eight hours of rest between training sessions is the minimum recommendation for recovery, with one study showing full recovery after 72 hours[2, 10, 20, 22]. Although most resistance training would require more rest it is likely that you could train your midsection every other day with little concern of overtraining.

Many of the muscles around our spine and trunk, and those smaller muscles that support our joints (i.e. our rotator cuff muscles in the shoulder), are comprised of muscle tissue more apt to endurance than strength and power. These muscles are often termed postural muscles because of their importance in maintaining optimal postural alignment against the force of gravity. Gravity being a constant, these muscles are stressed almost all the time. This may affect the optimal training frequency for core musculature, and the amount of rest required between sessions.

New ways to challenge your midsection:

Many individuals focus on how much they can lift. However, there is more to strength training than just lifting heavier weights. The body works as a system and must utilize groups of muscles to perform even the simplest tasks. You can ensure more core activity and improve the efficiency of these muscle groupings by performing exercises that challenge your balance and coordination. Studies have shown that performing exercises on a stability ball, or performing exercises with one arm or leg at a time, increased core activity and increased muscle recruitment in the surrounding musculature[6, 8, 13, 47]. For example, performing leg extensions (an exercise for the front of your thighs) while seated on a ball increases core and hamstring activity[6].

88

Try the following strategy to improve your upper body strength, coordination, and increase your core activity during your weight training sessions. First, ensure that you are performing exercises with good form, at a slow controlled tempo, and can keep your deep core muscles active by holding your belly button in for the entire set. You can use this progression during any cable, dumbbell, or band exercise. Change should be made every couple of weeks as you take the time to perfect your technique.

1. Both arms at the same time.
2. Alternating arms. (Note: you perform one complete rep with the left arm and then complete a rep with the right, but there is still weight in both hands.)
3. One arm at a time. (Note: you only have weight in one hand. Place the other hand on your hip and ensure that you do not twist or bend at the waist.)
4. Return to step one with heavier weights and repeat.

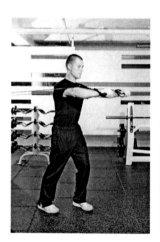 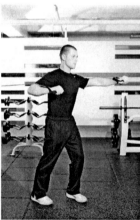 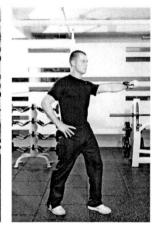

When you progress, challenge yourself to finish the same number of reps as you did before. If you continue to perfect your technique and increase your rep range, when you return to performing that exercise with both hands, you will be able to lift more weight, and have a stronger midsection to boot.

Other ways to challenge your stability and increase core activity include:

- progressing from machines, to cables, and then free weight exercise;
- performing exercises on one foot;
- performing seated and lying exercises on a Bosu ball or stability ball; or
- performing exercises on foam pads, half foam rolls, and balance boards

You can find many of these items at your local gym or purchase them online for home use at www.Performbetter.com.

Core exercise and lower back pain:

Evidence is building to show a relationship between weak core musculature, poor posture, and the incidence of low back pain[12, 22, 25]. It is likely that increasing core strength will improve your symptoms, but certain precautions must be followed:

- When injured, it is important to follow a progression of treatment starting with an orthopedic physician, followed by physical therapy, and finally work with a qualified fitness professional to modify your existing workout plan.
- Only perform exercises that do not cause further pain unless under the supervision of a medical professional.
- Stay away from leg raises, hanging leg raises, roman chair leg raises, leg lifts, bicycle kicks, ball and wheel roll-outs and those exercises that lock your feet into position. Studies have reported those exercises that involve leg movement and those that lock the feet into position increase the activity of hip flexor musculature and decrease the activity of abdominal musculature[15, 18]. Over-development of your hip flexor musculature may reduce hip flexibility, create posture problems,

increase shear forces on the lumbar vertebrae, and therefore increase low back pain.

- Unless prescribed by a physician stay away from weight belts and lumbar support devices. Studies show that lumbar support devices such as weight belts and cradles only increase lower back muscle activity[3, 35]. The National Strength and Conditioning Association only recommend using weight belts when performing lifts at near maximal loads[2]. Lifting of this intensity would be contraindicated for any individual with low back pain.
- For the reduction of low back pain, stabilization exercises may be more appropriate than exercises that involve movement. Generally, stabilization exercises are those that require static positions to be held for as long as possible, and exercises in which the goal is better balance and coordination. With these exercises, increased endurance and better form are your best markers of improvement. Activities like the bridge, side bridge, plank, quadruped, "super-mans", and cobras are great examples. Many of these exercises increase intensity by adding balls, or disks to create instability.
- Strength is not enough. A flexibility program is essential to recovering from low back pain. Focus on hip and low back flexibility as studies show a decrease in flexibility of this musculature is a precursor to low back pain[22].

SECTION III:
HOW TO GET PHYSICAL

Chapter 6:
Weight Training

Weight training became a popular topic as Arnold Schwarzenegger gained popularity winning Mr. Olympia and starring in classic films like *Pumping Iron, Conan,* and *Hercules in New York.* However, this topic is shrouded in myth. Advice on weight training has been based on tips from peers, genetically gifted sports heroes, your friendly neighborhood muscle-head, and magazines biased by the endorsement of supplement manufacturers. This is a far cry from peer-reviewed scientific literature and carefully planned research studies. Although body building is a catalyst that changed fitness training forever, science must be the driving force behind a more fit future. The benefits of resistance training extend to all populations, and new research has made improving your physique, getting healthier, and growing stronger easier than ever.

Myth #35: *You should only lift weights if you want to get big.*
What You Should Know: Everyone can benefit from strength training.

Although more and more people enter the weight room and benefit from resistance training, there is still a lingering stigma that only bodybuilders need to lift weights. Muscle is essential to function, enhances sports performance, and adding muscle mass enhances our appearance. It is what is responsible for giving us the "toned" or "more defined" look that has become so coveted. Some of us started really skinny and just wanted to rid ourselves of nicknames like "bean-pole" and "pipe-snake". I was one of these individuals. I started high school six feet tall and 145 pounds. I looked like a model; a female runway model that is. I could have played the part of every scrawny kid who got sand kicked in his face at the beach.

For those worried about getting "bulky" know that it is difficult to put on large amounts of muscle mass. Although our bodies add muscle mass in response to resistance training, only a finite amount of muscle tissue is created after a single weight lifting session. It is unlikely that you will get big by accident. Bodybuilders train hard for years to attain the large amount of muscle mass associated with their sport.

Myth #36: *Muscle turns into fat when you stop working out.*
What You Should Know: It's not physiologically possible.

Muscle cannot turn into fat. It just doesn't work that way. Muscle and fat are made of different stuff. However, studies have shown that when individuals reduce their physical activity it is not usually matched by a reduction in calories[67]. So when very muscular athletes become overweight, it is usually because they stop working out, but continue to consume the same amount of food as they did when playing sports. This creates a scenario in which one is consuming more calories than they burn. A calorie surplus will inevitably lead to an increase in fat storage.

The Benefits of Resistance Training – Something for Everyone

- **Increased Metabolism:** Research by Dr. Wayne Wescott, director of research for the YMCA, suggests that just one pound of muscle will burn as much as 35 calories per day at rest. *That's more calories being burned while you're sitting on your ass!!!*
- **Increased Muscle Mass:** Increased muscle mass is one way our body responds to the stress of resistance training, enhancing our appearance and increasing strength.

- **Decreased Risk of Heart Disease:** Heart disease is the leading cause of premature death in the United States[29].
- **Lower Cholesterol:** Adding a resistance training program to your exercise routine has been shown to improve cholesterol levels, specifically lowering LDL-C[35, 59]. Resistance training combined with cardio has been shown to be more effective at improving cholesterol then cardio alone.
- **Lower Blood Pressure:** Resistance training combined with a cardio program is an effective way to decrease your resting blood pressure, reducing your risk of coronary artery disease[65].
- **Increased Bone Density:** Just as your muscles adapt and increase in size and strength to handle larger amounts of weight, your bones increase in density to handle the new loads placed on your skeletal system[53]. This increase in bone density may reduce your risk of osteoporosis[29].
- **Decreased Risk of Various Types of Cancer:** The American College of Sports Medicine released a study in 2001, establishing a relationship between increased physical activity (duration and frequency) and a decreased risk of breast cancer[3]... *and that's just one example.*
- **Improved Mental Health:** Strength training has been shown to be very effective at improving mental health, especially depression. In a study at Harvard University, 10 weeks of strength training reduced clinical depression symptoms more successfully than standard counseling. In a study at Duke University, patients with major depression randomized to an exercise group had declines in depression equal to those on antidepressants, and exercisers were less likely to relapse 6 months later than the medicated group. In a study that tested the self satisfaction of college females, those who trained 2 and 3 days per week were more satisfied and had a better self concept[10].
- **Increased Physical Functioning:** Resistance training will make daily tasks easier - such as mowing the lawn, taking out the trash, or walking up a flight of stairs.

- **Improved Resting Insulin Levels and Increased Sensitivity[17, 28]:** In English… You decrease your risk of Type II Diabetes, the third largest cause of death in the United States. Although there are strong genetic ties with this disease, a sedentary lifestyle and obesity are primary contributing factors to its onset[29].
- **Improved Performance:** Whether you are a weekend warrior or a professional athlete, resistance training can have a huge impact on your performance. *Note: The type of resistance training used should become more "sports-specific" as your training becomes more advanced.*

How much resistance training do you need?

The amount of resistance training necessary will increase as your goals increase in difficulty and magnitude. With that being said, *anything is better than nothing.* Several studies have shown that just one session per week may increase strength[1, 12, 13, 40, 50, 61].

Use the following graph to help create general guidelines in your program based on your desired result.

Training Volume Continuum				
Conditioning	Days/Week	Time/Day	Sets/Muscle	Exercises/Session
Deconditioned	0	0	0	0
Better Health	1	30 min.	1	5-8
	1-2	45 min.	1-2	6-9
Fitness	2-3	60 min.	2-3	8-10
	3-4	90 min	3-4	9-12
Optimal Performance	4-5	2 hours	3-6	10-15
Elite Athlete	5+	2+ hours	3-8	2 sessions/day

Graph constructed using the following research and guidelines[1-3,5,10,13-15,19,23,25,33,40,47,52,56,63-64].

Myth #37: *More is always better.*
What You Should Know: You can have too much of a good thing.

More training will likely produce better results, but there is a limit[5, 13, 22, 26, 40, 55]. For those individuals who have made the commitment and desire optimal results: more work does not always equal better results. A study comparing Division 1 college athletes in an off-season training program compared three, four, five, and six day per week programs. The four and five day groups showed the largest improvement[26]. There is also evidence that suggests that we will likely recover slower as we age reducing the amount of training we are capable of[28, 42].

Interesting Tidbits: Research shows that the frequency of training may be more important than the volume of work in each session. A study divided previously untrained individuals into two groups. The first group performed three sets of eight exercises once a week. The second group engaged in one set of eight exercises three days a week. While both groups experienced strength gains, the second group had significantly larger improvements in strength[40].

How much rest do I need between weight training sessions?

At least one day of rest before working similar muscle groups again, but not more than three days of rest between sessions stressing similar muscle groups[2, 5, 21]. It is a generally accepted practice not to work muscles that are sore or feel tired from a previous workout. Resistance training affects muscular, hormonal, and neuromuscular systems causing fatigue. This requires a minimum of 48 hours for recovery with full recovery seen in 72 to 96 hours after exercise[7-8, 42, 46]. Factors that will influence recovery include the intensity and volume of training, training experience, and age[42, 46, 51]. You want to allow enough time to recover fully, but not allow too much time to pass resulting in a loss of the gains you made. Two to three sessions a week for similar musculature is ideal.

Myth #38: *Work each muscle group once a week.*
What You Should Know: Twice a week is better.

This common practice is not the most effective way to train. In a study on men with resistance training experience, the largest augmentation in strength happened after just three days of rest[62]. That means if you want to get the most out of your program, you should work each muscle every four days. Twice a week is a far more effective way to train than the one day per week program sometimes promoted by bodybuilding magazines.

Myth #39: *Three sets per exercise is the best way to train*
What You Should Know: There is no magic number.

Why do so many routines in magazines have you perform three sets of three different exercises for each muscle group? Is that really necessary? This 3 x 3 model has been handed-down by our fitness forefathers and is still used by many of the bodybuilders that grace the pages of weightlifting magazines. However, this is not the best way for a normal person to gain muscle. I say "normal" because there are several factors that allow bodybuilders to make gains from such an extreme regimen, and some of these factors are not "natural".

The American College of Sports Medicine recommends a minimum of one set of 8 to10 exercises stressing all the major muscle groups of the body for 8-12 repetitions, done twice a week (10 to 15 repetitions with lighter weight for an older population)[2]. These are guidelines for the novice exerciser and are much more appropriate for someone who is just getting started.

100

"Single set workouts versus multiple set workouts" has become a debate in the fitness industry over the past decade. However, I am not sure why. It is not a question of which is better, but which is appropriate for the beginner, and which is appropriate for the experienced lifter. When you are trying to make gains, you need to increase the number of sets you do per exercise, or increase the number of sets per muscle group in a progressive manner[5, 25].

Novice Lifter:

- Up to 16 weeks of training one set per exercise elicits similar results as multiple sets[47, 64].
- After 16 weeks of training, multiple sets are superior[19, 52]. (However, why not start with 2, once you have adapted to the new volume you can progress to 3, etc.)

Experienced Lifter:

- One set per exercise is inferior to multiple sets per exercise. In fact, this volume of training may not even be enough to maintain strength gains acquired from previous higher volume training[33, 45]. Note: Six sets per muscle group is the limit. More sets will not cause further improvement[13, 42].

The research supporting single set training only supports the notion for the previously untrained individual, after 16 weeks of training it is suggested that a multiple-set program be adopted. After 16 weeks, adopt a program of two sets per muscle. So many people jump straight to three sets, but why? In our fast paced society many individuals find it challenging to make time for the gym. If you can get results from a one or two sets per muscle group program, don't waste your time doing unnecessary work. If time is not an issue for you, than spend the extra time doing core training, stretching, or cardio.

There is a limit to the benefit that can be gained by simply adding more sets. In a series of studies little difference was found in strength (measured by number of repetitions) gained between three sets and seven sets of endurance type (higher reps with lower weight) resistance training[42].

How much rest do I need between sets?

The amount of rest between sets of exercise will vary depending on the load used and the intensity of your routine. Sets performed with lighter weights will generally require less recovery time than those sets performed with larger loads, explosive speeds, or done with high intensity. Other factors that will contribute to the selection of rest intervals include: training experience, conditioning, individual recoverability, nutritional status, and muscle mass utilized[5, 13].

Examples:
- Those just starting a routine will likely need more rest between sets than experienced lifters.
- Larger rest intervals may be required for exercises that use more muscle. For example, a squat will require more rest than a leg extension.
- The better you eat, the faster you can recover.

Rest Between Sets: General recommendations based on goal[4-6, 13, 49]

Training Goal (number of repetitions per set)	Rest period between sets for similar muscles
Endurance (12-25 Reps)	60 seconds or less
General Strength (8-12 Reps)	30-90 seconds
Hypertrophy (Growth) (8-12 Reps)	30-90 seconds
Maximal Strength (1-5 Reps)	2-3 minutes
Power/Explosiveness (1-5 Reps)	3-5minutes

What is The Best Range of Motion (ROM) for an Exercise?

Exercises should be performed through the largest range of motion that is comfortable, pain free, and can be done with good form[5, 13, 21, 25]. In general, as the load and/or speed of movement increases, the safe and/or comfortable range of motion will decrease.

The load being lifted, speed of movement, your level of flexibility, and the purpose of your training will determine your optimal range of motion.

- If your goal is increased strength, range of motion may be limited to decrease the risk of injury, and ensure proper form during heavy lifting. In a study comparing partial versus full ROM on the bench press, both elicited similar gains in maximal strength[38].
- ROM should be specific to the activity for which one is training[44]. If your training to increase your vertical jump and are utilizing exercises such as box jumps, depth jumps, and plyometric activity there is likely no need to deep squat with each jump, as this is not the most efficient way to jump.
- Injury often causes pain through certain ranges of motion and limits flexibility. It would be counter-productive to work through the pain and force your body through a range of motion that is restricted by the tightness caused from injury. In cases of injury please consult an orthopedic physician or physical therapist.
- Those activities performed with lighter weights at controlled tempos should utilize larger ranges of motion (ROM) to increase strength through your complete ROM. This may prevent further decreases in range of motion sometimes associated with resistance training.

Interesting Tidbits: If a full ROM is not utilized at a joint, soft tissues (tendons, ligaments, muscles) may compensate by shortening, further limiting your flexibility[5, 7, 21]. "If you don't use it, you lose it". Note that decreases in flexibility can lead to unhealthy joint mechanics in the ankle, knee, hip, and low back which may in turn lead to injury[13, 25].

Common Questions:

Q: When I do a bench press should I allow the bar to touch my chest, or should I stop when I reach 90 degrees at the elbow?
A: Go as far as you can comfortably go while maintaining good form.
Q: Should I do squats as deeply as I can, or should I stop when my upper leg reaches parallel with the floor?
A: Go as far as you can comfortably go while maintaining good form. As you increase your training loads and reduce reps your comfortable ROM will likely decrease. Note: I have met many individuals who could not perform a bodyweight squat with good form descending just a few inches. In this case flexibility training may be more important than additional weight.

Myth #40: *Heavier weight is always better.*
What You Should Know: The amount of weight you use (and the speed you move it) will depend on your goal[31].

We'll find the appropriate weight for your training by selecting a weight that will cause temporary muscular fatigue ("failure") within a repetition range that is appropriate for your goal. For example, if you want to put on more muscle then it is suggested you perform sets of 6 to 12 repetitions. This implies you need to find a weight that you can lift at least 6 times, but not more than 12 times. If you can do more than 12 repetitions you need to increase the weight, if you cannot do 6 repetitions with good form than you need to decrease the weight.

The speed with which you lift a weight should be sport or goal specific[31]. General guidelines are slow controlled contractions for endurance, general strength, and hypertrophy training; tempo increases as more power and maximum strength are desired. Refer to the chart below.

Note: The heavy loads used for maximal strength training are to be lifted as fast as can be controlled; however, the weight may move slower than it did for endurance training. If an increase in power is desired, note that a relatively light load is suggested, the weight used must allow for ballistic tempos with an emphasis on form and speed.

Recommended Reps and Tempo:

Training Goal	Velocity/Speed
Endurance (12-25reps)	Slow
General Strength (8-12reps)	moderate
Hypertrophy (Growth) (6-12reps)	moderate
Maximal Strength (1-6reps)	As fast as you can with control
Power (Neural) (1-6reps)	Explosive

Interesting tidbit: In a study, novice weight lifters were allowed to select weights they thought would improve their muscular strength on various pieces of equipment. The group selected weights that were too light to induce any gain in strength or size[66]. I would hate to see any individual waste their time with activities that would be ineffective for reaching their goal.

Is there an order I should do my exercises in?

In a study on the effects of exercise order and performance, those exercises performed at the end of a routine were done with fewer repetitions[55]. Prioritize your exercise accordingly.

It has been suggested by the National Academy of Sports Medicine that your core routine (trunk stabilization, axe chops, and crunches) precedes other strength training. Starting a routine with these exercises will "excite" core musculature so that they fire more effectively throughout your workout. "High levels of core strength improve segmental stabilization throughout the lumbo-pelvic-hip complex, which improves functional strength and neuromuscular efficiency of the entire kinetic chain."[13] Put simply, a strong core makes everything else stronger. After your core routine, move onto whole body exercises, which have the highest energy demand, followed by multi-joint movements, and then single joint movements[5].

Recommended order:

- Warm-Up
- Core
- Legs
- Back
- Chest
- Shoulder
- Arms
- Cardio
- Cool-down
- Stretch

For example: You may begin your workout with planks and crunches, followed by squats, then push-ups and rows, finishing your resistance training with curls and triceps extensions.

Split routine example: A chest workout could be standing cable chest (your entire body must stabilize the movement), followed by bench press, and finally flies.

Myth #41: *Split routines are more effective than whole body programs.*
What You Should Know: Split routines are simply over recommended.

Split routines split the body into different groups to be trained on separate days. This places an unrealistic demand on the individual with limited time. Optimal rest and frequency must be considered. The best results are achieved when strength training for each muscle group is done 2-3 times a week with 48 -72 hours rest between sessions. Even a three day split means being in the gym six days a week. A five day split simply allows too much rest before similar muscle groups are worked again.

Also, the muscular system works in an integrated fashion and should likely be trained as a system. For example, the muscles of your back, chest and shoulder all act to move the shoulder joint. Is it really appropriate to split those groups into separate days and potentially risk excessive wear on your shoulder joint and overtraining of your rotator cuff musculature?

Myth #42: *I work my legs when I do cardio, so I don't need to spend time lifting weights with my legs.*
What You Should Know: Cardio does very little to increase strength.

The body is an incredibly adaptable machine, but adaptation is specific. Cardio is a wonderful way to increase endurance, but is unlikely that cardio will increase leg strength, muscle mass, or create the chiseled legs you want. The overload that cardio creates is generally on our cardiovascular system, so the body adapts by preparing the cardiovascular system for an increase in activity with very little if any adaptation in muscular strength. The most effective means to increase muscle mass is resistance training. This includes freeweights, machines, bands, medicine balls, and in some exercises, the use of your own bodyweight or gravity as resistance. In a study of 35 male soldiers who performed either endurance training, resistance training, or a combination of both, only those who included lower body resistance training in their program increased leg strength[32].

Myth #43: *No Pain, No Gain.*
What You Should Know: That's Bull!

Two factors that keep a beginner from coming back to the gym: muscle soreness and the perception that resistance training must be hard to get results. You do not have to be sore to get results. In fact, constantly increasing the volume of your training to continually make yourself sore can lead to overtraining and a reduction in performance[13].

In two studies comparing the rate of perceived exertion and load, lower weights with higher reps were perceived as easier than training that involved the use of heavier weights with lower rep ranges[20, 34]. Lighter loads, those allowing 10 to 20 repetitions per set, are effective for creating gains in strength and muscle mass in beginners. Why not start your training routine with lighter loads and higher reps and slowly increase the weight as you become accustomed to resistance training?

Interesting Tidbit: Stretching, yoga, and proper cool-downs have been shown to be effective in reducing soreness (See the chapter "stretching stuff" for details).

Myth #44: *A new exercise will shock your muscles.*
What You Should Know: Muscles are stupid; they cannot differentiate between two similar exercises.

All a muscle can do is contract or shorten, usually pulling two bones closer together. They do not twist, bend, change shape (other than increase in size) or "tone up". With this in mind, the best exercise for any muscle is one that allows a muscle to contract through a full range of motion in opposition to some form of resistance. A muscle cannot differentiate between a band, a free weight, or your own body weight. In a study on muscle recruitment in the quadriceps (the big muscles on the front of your upper leg), there was no difference between squats and leg extensions. The squat caused the quads to contract harder, but this could have been a function of increased load[54]. Stay away from the idea of "shocking a muscle," and try to think big picture. Besides, shocking a muscle is really the "spot reduction myth" in disguise.

So why choose different exercises at all? Although a single muscle does not know the difference between two similar exercises, we can select exercises that will challenge our body to better coordinate various muscles. Your nervous system and other musculature become more involved when you choose more complex exercises (squats over leg extensions) or train in unstable environments (bands and free weights are more "unstable" than machines). The coordination of various muscles may enhance your performance and allow you to lift heavier weights, do more reps, or perform complex exercises that burn more calories.

Most importantly, choose the activities you enjoy. All exercise has its benefits and drawbacks, but results can only be realized if you do the exercise often enough and long enough to see results. The best exercise is the one you like and will do with frequency.

Myth #45: *Changing exercises will keep you from hitting a plateau.*
What You Should Know: Changing exercises is not enough.

If you want to continue seeing results, you need to change how your muscles pull, not what your muscles pull on. You need to change how much, how long, or how fast you are pulling. Change your rep range, the weight you use, the tempo at which you perform each repetition, or the very nature of your training to continue seeing results[1, 5, 12, 29]. Training programs that continually use the same load, intensity, rep range, and volume may lead to overuse injuries[13]. For a good example of this system put into practice, check out a typical program many bodybuilders utilize to continue seeing results:

- Moderate weight for 6-12 reps per set (Hypertrophy training), done for 4-8 weeks
- Light weight for 12 - 20 slow reps per set (Endurance training), done for 4-8 weeks
- Moderate weight for 6-12 reps per set (Hypertrophy training), done for 4-8 weeks
- Heavy weight for 1-6 reps per set (Max Strength Training), done for 4 weeks
- Repeat

This program allows a bodybuilder's muscles to get better at one aspect of muscular performance, but changes when a new adaptation is necessary to see further results.

Cross-training is another effective way to bust through plateau platitude. An example of cross training for a basketball player may include:

- Resistance training for strength
- Yoga for flexibility and balance
- Boxing for improved hand speed and coordination
- Basketball for continued skill development

Many athletes will utilize various types of training to improve their performance. The various methods of training give the body something new to adapt to.

More Programming Examples (Simple Periodization):

Four to eight weeks is recommended for each phase or type of training. Four weeks will give you the time you need to get good at the routine, make gains, and adapt to the training stimulus. Once the body has adapted to the routine (generally four-eight weeks in a phase) it is less likely that you will continue to make gains. This may be referred to as a "state of diminishing returns" - you will get less and less out of the same work load. This is when you change to a new training stimulus.

Weight Loss, and "Toning"

Program:

- Endurance Training for 4-8 weeks
- Strength Training for 4-6 weeks
- Endurance Training for 4 weeks
- Strength Training for 4 weeks
- Continue switching between Strength and Endurance training in 4 week blocks

Rationale:
The relative high rep range and short rest period between sets of endurance training creates a high volume of training, and therefore, burns a ton of calories. Your strength training will allow you to add moderate amounts of muscle mass to increase your resting metabolism.

Increased Muscle Mass

Program:

- Hypertrophy Training for 4 weeks
- Endurance Training for 4weeks
- Hypertrophy Training for 4 weeks
- Maximum Strength Training for 4 weeks

Repeat in 4 week blocks

Rationale:

The parameters for hypertrophy training are most effective for increasing muscle mass, but we have to continually create change. Increased endurance will help to keep your stabilization system strong and increase muscular endurance. When you return to hypertrophy training you should note that you can do more reps of the weight you were doing in your previous hypertrophy phase. Make sure you adjust the weight to stay within the recommended rep range. Switching to max strength will allow you to increase the loads you can lift through certain neural adaptations.

General Health:

Program:

Periodization for general health is similar to weight loss. Depending on your goals it may be necessary to add low level agility, and/or max strength loads to your routine. However, it is not suggested that those of you who workout for general health participate in the same type of power training, or the type of max strength phase that is routinely used by elite athletes.

Rationale:

An increase in muscular endurance, general strength, and muscle mass, will provide you with the health benefits listed previously and make daily life easier. Max Strength and Power Training may provide more risk than benefit for this group; however, it is important to train in preparation for life. Recreational sport, heavy lifting, and/or an active lifestyle may necessitate a need for a couple of low level power and/or whole body max strength exercises added to your routine.

Perform Better: Training for Sport:

Program:

- Endurance Training
- Hypertrophy Training
- Max Strength Training
- Power Training

Repeat emphasizing those phases that are most important to your sport or the ones in which you exhibit the most weakness.

Rationale:

Sports rely heavily on all types of strength. Each phase provides a different stimulus for muscular, hormonal, and neural systems. Each phase of training is interrelated and built on top of the other to create the highest levels of performance.

Goal Specific Recommendations (Summary) [2, 5, 13]

Training Goal	Reps/Set	Sets/Muscle	Velocity/Tempo	Rest Between Sets
Endurance	12 - 25	1-3	Slow	60 seconds or less
General Strength	8 - 12	1-5	Moderate	30-90 seconds
Hypertrophy (Growth)	8 - 12	1-5	Moderate	30-90 seconds
Maximal Strength	1 - 5	4-6	As fast as you can w/ control	2-3 minutes
Power (Neural Adaptation)	1 – 5	4-6	Explosive	3-5minutes

Note: Power training may refer to plyometrics, speed, and/or agility training.

Don't get discouraged:

Those who are just beginning a training routine may have dramatic gains in strength (up to 300% in the first three months), but see little change in their physique. The dramatic gains in strength in this initial stage of training are primarily changes in your neuromuscular system (your mind muscle connection)[5, 13]. Muscle growth starts in the early stages of training, but it may take four weeks for a measurable change in muscle mass[5]. Note that after three or four months of training, further increase in muscle strength are attributed to an increase in muscle mass[5, 25]. Unfortunately, there is no way to skip this step and start muscle growth immediately. So keep training!!!

Myth #46: *If you want to lose weight…. Start with lots of cardio. Weight training will just make you big.*

What You Should Know: Weight training is a powerful weight loss tool.

Resistance training can impact weight loss in 3 significant ways:
1. Resistance training burns calories[9]. The more reps, sets, and weight you do, the more calories you will burn.
2. Resistance training creates a post exercise increase in metabolism[9, 11, 16, 43]. Your body must burn calories to repair body tissues and make changes to prepare you for your next session.
3. Weight training can increase your resting metabolism. The more muscle you have, the more calories you burn.

Interesting Tidbits: A combination of resistance training and cardio may create a larger decrease in body fat than cardio alone. Researchers from Dong-A University in Korea, and the University of Tokyo, compared the effects of no training, resistance training and cardio training together, and cardio training alone in middle aged women in a 24 week program. The researchers found that the combined group had the largest decrease in abdominal fat, and were the only group to have a significant increase in lean body mass [25].

The rise in metabolism following exercise is often referred to as E.P.O.C. (Excess Post Exercise Oxygen Consumption). Resistance training creates a larger increase in "E.P.O.C." than aerobic activity when matched for oxygen consumption and duration[11, 16]. When resistance training and cardiovascular activity were performed in a single session E.P.O.C. was greater than resistance training or cardio training alone[16].

The Gender Gap:

The differences between how men and women respond to resistance training is relatively small. Although it is likely that women will not grow as much muscle and may carry more body fat, the improvements that women can make with resistance training are similar to their male counterparts[36]. I have witnessed many females out perform their male counterparts with a little dedication and hard work.

The "Benefits of Resistance Training" (chart on pages 82-84) are not limited to men, nor should resistance training be thought of as men's activity. A study of 16 weeks of resistance training in young women found moderate load resistance training caused positive adaptations in both bone density and muscle mass, decreasing the risk of osteoporosis[53]. In a study performed by Westcott and his colleagues the average woman who strength trained, gained 1.75 pounds of lean weight, but lost 3.5 pounds of fat over an 8 week period.

Possibly, the biggest disservice in the fitness industry is the marketing strategy towards women. Many media sources geared towards women perpetuate the "toning" and "spot reduction" myths. I still see countless women trying to target their inner thighs or tone up the back of their arms. Working small areas burns a small amount of calories. Put simply ladies, the soft stuff is usually fat, and will only decrease when the amount of calories you take in, is less than the calories you burn. Concentrate on larger, multi-joint movements, such as chest press, rows and squats. These exercises incorporate more muscles including your trouble areas, and they will help you burn more calories.

More disturbing is the advertisements, whether intentional or non-intentional, that have created a notion in our society that women should exhibit the same leanness as their pre-pubescent counterparts. Every time I pick up a magazine there is some gaunt model on the cover, void of essential fat and in many cases void of any significant muscle. Remember, fat is there for a reason and serves many important functions in the body. 18 to 23 percent body fat is a healthy range for a female. Many women on the cover of many magazines are so far below the norm that they may be deemed unhealthy.

The American College of Sports Medicine warned the athletic community of something known as the female athlete triad, in which the obsession with leanness causes women to heavily restrict caloric intake and/or workout excessively. This leads to disordered eating patterns, abnormal hormone secretion disrupting the menstrual cycle (oligomenorrhea, amenorrhea), and because estrogen is essential in maintaining strong bones in women this further leads to decreased bone density possibly causing a premature and/or severe onset of osteoporosis[25]. Unfortunately in my career I see this pattern reaching young women in all walks of life. If our goal is health, where did we take a wrong turn? I understand that we can be a very vanity driven society but health must precede all other goals.

Chapter 7:
Clearing Up Cardio Confusion

Public awareness and education concerning cardiovascular exercise seems to be better than the other forms of exercises discussed in this book. However, I still find myself lying awake at night wondering why more people don't participate. Cardio has several advantages over other forms of exercise: there are plenty of activities to choose from, everyone can participate in some form of cardio, cardio can be done almost anywhere, and the benefits of cardio are well-researched and documented.

> **Myth #47:** *I'm young, I don't need cardio.*
> **What You Should Know:** Young and unfit, could lead to old and fat.

Studies have examined the decreasing level of youth fitness and the increased risk of cardiovascular disease in various races, and ethnic groups[39, 47-48, 56, 57, 67, 84, 87, 133]. A lack of aerobic and physical fitness in adolescence has shown a strong correlation to adult fatness[129, 133]. Skipping out on your cardio is creating a bad habit that will eventually come back to haunt you. As your body fat slowly increases and/or your fitness level slowly decreases your chances of premature death steadily climb.

Why should I do cardio?

There are a multitude of benefits associated with cardiovascular exercise. Individuals of every age, regardless of their goal, have something to gain from it. Cardio is truly an essential component of a well planned exercise program.

Reduced body fat and/or weight loss:

The most time efficient way to burn calories, cardio has a powerful impact on our weight loss goals. The more calories you burn, the more fat you lose. Note: Research suggests that cardiovascular activity should be done a minimum of three days a week to reduce subcutaneous body fat[1, 20, 100-101, 104].

Decreased risk of cardiovascular disease, and premature death[15, 70-71, 74, 83, 86, 98, 104]:

Heart Disease: Several health factors are associated with an increased risk of heart disease, many of which can be improved upon with cardio.

- High blood pressure[10, 95, 122]
- High cholesterol[28]
- HDL/LDL Ratio[69]
- High triglycerides[69]
- High resting heart rate[92, 122]
- Elevated C-reactive protein[42, 78, 97]
- Hyperinsulinemia (precursor to, sign, and/or symptom of diabetes)
- Being overweight[26, 47, 49]
- Sedentary lifestyle, physical inactivity[70]
- Poor cardiovascular fitness[86]

Decreased risk of diabetes:

- Cardiovascular exercise improves glucose tolerance and insulin sensitivity decreasing the risk of Type II Diabetes[8, 31, 32].

Decreased risk of cancer:

- Exercise may play a protective role against various types of cancer. Studies show that the more you exercise the less risk you have of developing breast and colon cancers. In studies on various other cancers, including endothelial, ovarian, rectal, prostate, testicular, and lung cancers, research has noted a tendency towards reduced risk with 3 to 4 hours of moderate to intense physical activity per week[125].

Better Mental Health

- *Stress relief:* Cardio may be the secret to coping with stress. One study showed cardio to be better for recovery from stress than stress management education[118]. Physiologically cardio decreases the rise in blood pressure associated with the response to a stressful situations[5].

- *Relief from depression:* Exercise has a positive effect on mental health, and cardio is no exception. Several studies have shown that cardiovascular exercise may be an effective method for reducing symptoms of major depression[35-36, 81].

Fewer days missed from work:

- Research shows a reduction in absenteeism from work with just one day of exercise per week. Those who exercised twice a week or more missed fewer days[63].

Improved bone and joint health.

- **Less back pain:** Cardiovascular exercise may help to prevent instances of low back pain by preventing the deconditioning of low back musculature[131].

- **Less arthritis pain:** Osteoarthritis can be a debilitating disease. Often osteoarthritis reduces the amount of physical activity an individual participates in, leading to decreased fitness and weight gain. One study even linked arthritis with an increased risk of cardiovascular disease[75]. However, another study revealed that cardiovascular exercise done as little as 3 times per week for 25 minutes greatly decreased the amount of overall pain[131]. Less pain could mean better function, more activity, and better health.

- **Decreased risk of osteoporosis:** As we age our bone mineral density decreases making bones weak and fragile. Cardiovascular exercise increases peak bone density during youth, maintains bone density through adulthood, and reduces the amount of bone mineral loss during our later years. This is especially true of weight bearing activities. Weight bearing activities are those exercises that require you to support your body weight (cardio done in a standing position). Examples include: running, elliptical trainers, stairmasters, and most sporting activities. Although research has not been able to determine an ideal frequency of exercise, it does appear that it takes less exercise to maintain bone mineral density, than it does to increase it[12, 131].

Perform Better:

- **Play harder:** All exercise, regardless of the duration and/or intensity must utilize the cardio-respiratory system to sustain activity and/or recuperate from it[27]. A well-conditioned cardio-vascular system will enable you to play harder and longer.

- **Recover faster:** Cardiovascular exercise will improve recovery time from oxygen debt and a return to your resting heart rate[18]. Even if your sport is a short duration event such as sprinting, power lifting, baseball, or bodybuilding, cardiovascular exercise will improve recovery time increasing the productivity of your training. The shorter recovery time between sets means more work done in the same amount of time. This allows for better preparation before competition.

Myth #48: *If I can't get in 3 days this week, why bother?*
What You Should Know: Every bit counts.

Do not give up on your training because this week, you cannot get to the gym as often as you would like. Scheduling conflicts will arise, and maintaining your cardiovascular fitness can be achieved with less work. Significant detraining from endurance activities happens in just 12 days [52]. You can maintain your conditioning even by reducing frequency by 1/3 or even 2/3 as long as intensity of your cardio is maintained[13]. Even one good day in a tough week can prevent you from taking a step backwards. At the very least, a reduction in performance can be decreased by continuing your exercise program in whatever fashion your schedule allows[18].

The American College of Sports Medicine (ACSM) has been at the forefront of the health and fitness industry, establishing the minimum guidelines for exercise for more than 50 years. The following guidelines were established by the hard work of dedicated professionals using the latest in exercise research.

How Often?

- Between three and five times a week seems to be the optimal frequency for cardiovascular exercise. (Example: work-out a day, rest a day). Anything less than three days a week makes weight loss goals difficult to achieve[1, 20, 100-101, 104]. Less cardio-vascular training may result in improvements, but usually a higher intensity is required. Doing more than five days a week of cardiovascular activity may not provide any additional ben-efit, and your risk of injury increases disproportionately[52].

How Long?

• Cardio should be performed for 20 to 60 minutes (excluding warm-up and cool-down). This can be completed in one con-tinuous bout or intermittent bouts of at least 10 minutes in length accumulated throughout the day. As the intensity of your cardiovascular program increases to high or very high levels the duration of the activity will decrease to 20 - 30 min-utes a day and may be done in shorter 4 - 6 minute bouts[6].

How Hard?

• ACSM recommends moderate intensity programs with longer durations for most adults. This recommendation is made real-izing that a high proportion of adults are sedentary with at least one cardiovascular risk factor. Moderate intensity pro-grams should elicit significant results while reducing the risk associated with high intensity programs[13].

• High intensity exercise is recommended for sport specific goals, and for improving the performance of advanced exercisers.

What Type?

• Try to find activity you enjoy. There are plenty of options. Choosing an activity that you hate will likely result in a failure to comply with the recommended frequency and duration, but the best cardio exercises utilize your largest muscles in a rhythmic fashion. Good examples include, cardio machines, classes, walking or running outdoors, field sports, tennis and swimming.

Myth #49: _____ *is the best cardio*
What You Should Know: The best cardio is the cardio you like.

A real conversation I had with a gym member:
Brent: So, what's your goal?
Member: I want to lose a few pounds?
Brent: What have you done to start increasing the amount of calories you burn?
Member: Cardio.
Brent: What type?
Member: I run.
Brent: How long and how often do you run?
Member: A couple of times a week, for like 20 minutes at a time.
Brent: But, I see you at the gym five days a week. Why don't you run more often, and speed up your weight loss.
Member: Because I hate to run.
Brent: So why do you run?
Member: I heard it burns the most calories.
Brent: It's true that running burns a lot of calories; however, if you chose an exercise you actually enjoy, and did 30 minutes every time you come to the gym you could virtually pick any piece of equipment in the gym and burn more calories.
Member: I never thought about that.
Brent: So, what do you like?
Member: Ben and Jerry's.
Brent: OK, how about cardio?
Member: I really like classes. The elliptical trainer is cool, and I don't mind reading on my exercise bike at home.

Brent: Great, sounds like a plan. You can do classes when they fit into your schedule, the elliptical trainer on days they don't, and do the exercise bike on the weekends while you read the paper. Let me know how much weight you lose in the next couple of weeks.

All exercise has its benefits and risks. When choosing the best cardio for *you* apply these 4 guidelines.

1. Find an activity you enjoy (or at least hate the least).
2. Start small and increase the intensity and duration of exercise as your fitness level improves.
3. Be creative, keep it fun, and change things up.
4. Cardiovascular exercise done for increased performance and/ or in preparation for sport must mimic your activity as closely as possible, especially as the season approaches (see "Cardio for athletes").

Myth #50: *Cardio is cardio, it all does the same thing.*
What You Should Know: Cardio should be goal specific and provide an appropriate level of challenge based on your training experience.

For Beginners:

Anything is better than nothing.

- 9000 steps or more per day is an effective way to improve cholesterol (HDL/LDL ratio) and triglyceride levels[69].
- Increased fitness was achieved in a group of beginners with as little as one hour per week, done all at once, or in three 20-minute sessions[91].
- Vigorous activity done for 60 minutes six times per MONTH decreased coronary risk factors[71].
- Brisk walking has been studied extensively, and has been proven effective in improving cardiovascular fitness in

beginners — even when bouts of walking are broken up in to several shorter sessions throughout the day[52, 90]. In fact, a study showed that three, 10-minute bouts of walking done five days a week was as effective as 30 minute sessions done five days per week for reducing body fat, decreasing coronary artery disease risk, and improving mood[90].

Interesting Tidbit: The ACSM and the Center of Disease Control and Prevention have promoted the "Exercise-Lite Program" for almost two decades now: "Light to moderate exercise done most, if not all, days of the week for a total of 30 minutes a day. Bouts can be broken into several shorter sessions of 8-10 minutes[52]." This program is great for those starting an exercise program, and is based on a comprehensive review of research examining the amount of exercise required for a substantial decrease in morbidity rate (premature death). What are you waiting for? Get up; take a walk around the block, and when you get back you will be half way to 30 minutes.

For Intermediate:

You can expect better results if you do cardio more often, at a higher intensity, and/or increase the duration of exercise per session[58, 70, 74, 93].

A couple of examples:

- Those who took more than 8000 steps per day were 65% less likely to develop hypertension than those who walked less than 4000 steps a day, as well those who exercised more than three times per week showed significantly lower risk of disease than those who worked out less than three times per week[58].
- The more active you are, the less likely you are to suffer from premature death. Weekly physical activity resulting in 1000 calories burned reduces all cause morbidity by 20-30%[74].

For Advanced:

Being the best takes dedication; enhancing athletic performance often requires a larger amount of cardio than what is recommended for general health and fitness. Three or more days of cardio a week at a moderate to high intensity is likely the minimum cardio required for an increase in sports performance[113, 114].

The type of cardio you select should mimic your sport as closely as possible. Your body is so amazing at adaptation that it will literally make you better at the specific action you utilized during training while showing little sign of improvement in other activities. For example, an Olympic long distance swimmer, may be in great cardiovascular shape, but not be able to keep up with a recreational runner. The opposite is also true. You may be able to run for miles, but not last more than a few laps in a pool. Several studies have demonstrated that adaptations to various modes of cardiovascular activity are specific to that activity[61, 89].

Ideas for training:

- Field sports may benefit from high intensity interval training on a treadmill.
- Cross country skiers may utilize a hill program on an elliptical trainer with arms, set at a high level of resistance.
- Competitive cyclists will likely gain little from a running program on a treadmill, but may use spin classes in the gym during the colder winter months.

Common Cardio Questions:

I do cardio every day, but the boxing class at my club kills me. Why is boxing so hard?

Studies show that heart rate response is significantly higher for arm exercise versus leg exercise at the same workload[52]. The increased heart rate would definitely have an effect on how you feel. Studies also show that there is very little crossover between trained and untrained limbs in response to cardio[52]. In other words, running on a treadmill which works primarily your legs will have little effect on your performance in a boxing class which is predominately arms.

I run miles every day but can't swim three laps in a pool. Why is swimming so hard?

When swimming you hold your breath between strokes reducing the amount of oxygen you take in. Your body has to utilize oxygen to produce more energy, for your working muscles. Less available energy means fatigue is going to approach much faster than activities in which you can breathe normally. Some of the difficulty is also associated with what is termed a "training effect". If you do not practice all the time, chances are you are a pretty inefficient swimmer.

Interesting Tidbits:
- Several studies have noted discrepancies in intensity between practice and competitive game play[119, 139]. Although the early part of your off-season can be used for much needed rest, it is important to stay focused as the season approaches and keep your intensity high.
- When planning your cardio program, try to find a balance between enough and too much. Take notes and track the results from your training program to ensure that you have found that balance. Doing cardio more than five times a week will result in little or no improvement and increase your risk of injury disproportionately[13]. Increasing the amount of time and intensity per day improved performance up to a certain point, and then any further increase in volume decreased performance, possibly signaling overtraining[23].

Myth #51: *Doing cardiovascular exercise will burn up all my muscle.*
What You Should Know: Cardio does not burn muscle it burns sugar and fat.

Studies show that when cardio is added to a weight lifting program there is no decrease in gains[29, 60, 138]. In essence the addition of cardiovascular activity to the program did not take away from the resistance training program.

Muscles are composed of proteins, and your body would rather not use protein for fuel. Generally, your body gets between 3 - 5% of its energy from protein. Even during prolonged exhaustive events such as an ultra-marathon, the energy contributed by protein is not likely to exceed 15-18 percent[18, 40, 52]. On a side note, low carb diets are likely to increase the body's breakdown of protein for fuel, and many recreational lifters use these diets. These diets are not appropriate for an exercise population[40].

In a possible plus for strength athletes and bodybuilders, studies show a significant increase in growth hormone and testosterone released post cardiovascular activity[29, 54]. Both hormones play substantial roles in muscle growth[18].

Myth #52: *Nasal strips improve cardiovascular performance and/or recovery by opening nasal passages and allowing more air into the lungs.*
What You Should Know: Using nasal strips will not help you take in more air.

I have seen athletes from almost every sport wear nasal strips to improve their performance. Football players seem to be especially fond of this practice. In three separate studies, nasal strips had no effect on performance[24, 102, 124]. Practically speaking, if you need to get large volumes of air into your lungs, you are not going to breathe through your nose. When you get winded, don't you breathe through your mouth?

Myth #53: *I don't need cardio to get better at my sport.*

What You Should Know: Poker isn't a sport.

Unless the addition of Poker to ESPN-2 classifies this as a sport, I cannot think of a sporting activity that would not benefit from a cardiovascular program. All exercise, regardless of the duration and/or intensity must utilize the cardio-respiratory system to either sustain activity or recuperate from it[27]. Your cardiovascular system, like your muscular system, must be worked to maintain good health.

Cardio will:

- Decrease your risk of heart disease (this may not be sport specific, but it is long-life important);
- allow you to play harder, longer;
- reduce body fat, essentially, decreasing non-working mass;
- improve your recovery rate from intense activity; and
- even if your sport is a short duration event (sprinting, power lifting, baseball, bodybuilding), the shorter recovery time could increase the productivity of your training, allowing for better preparation before competition.

Myth #54: *Strength training can only hinder my cardiovascular performance.*
What You Should Know: Strength training could be the tool that propels your cardiovascular performance to new levels.

Just as cardiovascular fitness is essential to maintain or recover from any physical activity, a certain level of strength and/or power is essential to all movement. Even the amount of force required to propel someone a single step requires strength. If an individual could push off with more force or bring that next leg forward a faster, would that not make someone a little faster? This is clearly evident in a study that analyzed the mechanics of several runners at various speeds. As speed increased, the strength and length of muscle contractions in the butt muscles and hamstrings increased[73].

Some of the benefits endurance athletes can expect from adding a resistance training program:

- Increased Workload Capacity[59, 60]
  - o Train harder, longer
- Decreased Lactate Accumulation[59, 60]
  - o Increased lactic acid threshold, and decreased lactic acid accumulation increasing time to fatigue
- Decreased Post Training Fatigue[19]
  - o Feel better at the end of your training sessions
- Improved Running Economy[65]
  - o Improvements in running efficiency may help you set new personal bests
- Increased Force Output per Stroke/Step[73, 123]
  - o Get more out of every step

While not all of the benefits attained by adding a weight training routine to an endurance athletes program are well understood, several studies have shown improvement in endurance performance without an increase in aerobic capacity[19, 38, 59, 65]. That is, benefits were attained without an increase in your heart and lung's ability to perform. For those of you who have been training for quite some time, this is great news. As you know, it becomes harder and harder to make improvements in your performance the longer and harder you train. If you currently do a large volume of endurance training and have not seen results, adding strength training to your routine may be the ticket to a new level of performance. Max Strength and Power Training will likely have the largest effect on the performance of advanced endurance athletes[38]. However, there are various types of strength that may be addressed with specific strength training programs. Each type of strength training promotes various adaptations that may be beneficial for your endurance performance.

Strength-Endurance training: Weight training done with more repetitions per set (12-25), lower weights, a slow tempo, and often in a less stable environment. This training promotes stability, and the ability of your muscles to maintain strength for prolonged periods of time. This is the ideal starting point for those who are new to endurance training and/or resistance training[38, 121].

Strength training: This training involves heavier loads, with fewer reps per set and promotes an increase in your muscles ability to produce force. Many studies have shown a relationship between strength and performance in the endurance athlete[65, 73, 123].

Power training: This type of training usually incorporates sprinting, box jumps, power step-ups and medicine ball drills done at explosive tempos. This improves a muscles ability to generate force *quickly*. Power training has been shown to be an effective tool in improving running economy[128].

> **Myth #55:** *You will burn more fat by performing cardiovascular exercise at a lower intensity.*
> **What You Should Know:** To maximize your fat loss - work at the highest intensity you can comfortably maintain for the amount of time you wish to do cardio.

Doesn't it seem strange that you could burn more fat by working less? Doesn't it seem illogical to say walking on a treadmill is going to make you leaner than if you jogged? Both of these things sound strange because they're both wrong. This myth is so widespread, it is posted on most cardiovascular equipment (ex. cardio zone vs. fat burn zone), in personal training manuals, professional texts, and popular magazines. Despite this myths proliferation it remains an example of poorly interpreted research.

You do burn more fat at a lower intensity, but only as a *percentage* of the total calories burned. Although this concept is important to exercise professionals who must understand how the body fuels activity, it has little, if any, impact on your fat loss goals. In short, fat calories burned does not decrease as exercise intensity increases regardless of the change in percentage of fat utilized[62]. As exercise intensity increases, you simply burn more of both with sugar making up the largest percentage of calories. Would you rather have 50 percent of $100.00 or 20 percent of $500.00?

Make no mistake about it, if you only have 30 minutes to work out, higher intensity exercise will burn more calories from fat and sugar, which in turn reduces your fat storage. Research shows that to reduce body fat, cardiovascular activity should be done a minimum of three days a week, with an intensity and duration sufficient enough to burn 250-300 calories per session[1, 13, 20, 101, 104]. As physical activity increases, body fat will decrease. It is suggested that participants try to burn a minimum of 3500 calories per week (3500 calories = 1 pound of fat). 45 - 60 minutes of purposeful walking performed at a moderate intensity on most days of the week would accomplish this goal[107].

Interesting Tidbits: The higher your intensity is during your cardio session the more calories you will continue to burn post exercise[114].

Understanding how your body fuels activity:

Your body runs on a fuel mixture, much like a weed-wacker or snow-blower. It uses fat and sugar (and to a very small degree, protein) in various percentages to meet your body's energy needs. When you are at rest or working at lower intensities, your body uses a larger percentage of fat for fuel. As the intensity of exercise increases, your body utilizes more and more sugar to keep up with the increased demand for energy. With that being said, your body's fuel mixture is at its highest fat percentage at rest. That's right; you burn the most fat when you're lying in your bed, *but only as a percentage of calories burned.*

I think of fat like charcoal in a barbeque grill. It burns slow, efficiently, and there is a lot of it. However, they are hard to get started, they take a long time to heat up, and coals do not burn as hot. If we need extreme heat now, we have to add a fuel that is easier to burn. This is why sugar is important. Think of sugar like lighter fluid. Lighter fluid is required to start the coals, burns fast, burns extremely hot, but does not burn for nearly as long. Your body utilizes fat at lower intensities including rest to maintain biological function, replenish sugar stores, and handle low intensity activity. When you perform high intensity activities, your body burns a larger percentage of sugar to match the increased demand for energy.

How does this effect weight loss? Well, if you continually pour lighter fluid on charcoals, you will burn the charcoals down to the ground. Your body works in a similar fashion. Body fat reduction is dependent on creating a calorie deficit. Whether moving burns sugar or fat you will lose weight.

Interesting Tidbit: More fit could mean less fat: Fit individuals utilize similar percentages of fat and sugar to fuel activity as unfit individuals. But because fit individuals are able to maintain higher intensities, more calories are burned, both fat and sugar, in the same amount of time[62]. It's nice to know that as your fitness level improves it may get easier to stay lean.

Cardio recommendations for disease prevention:

Cholesterol: Improvements in blood lipid profile seem to favor volume over intensity. That is, the more often you do cardio, the better your improvements in cholesterol[83, 114]. One study showed 40 minutes of exercise per day, 3 days per week, improved HDL/LDL ratio significantly[28].

Cardiovascular disease: The more cardio you do the lower your risk of cardiovascular disease[70].

Cancer: The more you exercise the lower your risk of breast and colon cancers. Various other cancers including endothelial, ovarian, rectal, prostate, testicular, and lung cancers have also been studied. Research has noted a tendency towards reduced risk with 3 to 4 hours of moderate to intense physical activity per week[125].

Osteoporosis: Although research has not been able to determine an ideal frequency of exercise, reducing your risk of developing osteoporosis seems to favor higher intensity activities[114]. Examples include cardio done in a standing position: running, elliptical trainers, stair-masters, and most sporting activities. It does appear that it takes less exercise to maintain bone mineral density, than it does to increase it[12, 131].

Blood Pressure: Decreases in blood pressure seem to favor an increase in the total amount of cardio you do (length and frequency of sessions) over intensity[114]. In one study, 150 minutes of cardio per week done at a moderate intensity improved blood pressure within 3 to 6 months[94].

Type II Diabetes: Since the changes in glucose tolerance and insulin sensitivity usually deteriorate within 72 hours, doing cardio often is imperative. ACSM recommends a volume of exercise equivalent to 1000 calories burned per week[8]. Two studies have recommended intensity hard enough to induce a sweat when trying to decrease the risk of Type II Diabetes[114]. Try to do some cardiovascular activity every day.

Mental Health: Improved mental health seems to favor moderate intensity cardio over high intensity activity[114]. That is, doing cardiovascular activity at a comfortable pace will have a larger impact on your mental health.

Tips and Ideas for Optimizing Your Cardio Program:

Just be more active. As mentioned before, recreational activities (ex. gardening), vigorous physical activity (ex. sports), walking a slightly longer commute, or taking more than 9000 steps per day have all been linked to a decreased risk of cardiovascular disease[3, 31, 39, 53, 56, 57, 69, 104, 113, 129-130].

Brisk walking has been studied extensively and has been proven effective in improving cardiovascular fitness in beginners. This holds true even when bouts of walking are broken up into several shorter sessions throughout the day[52, 90].

Resistance training may improve cardiovascular fitness[44-46,111,126]. Circuit training, or doing various resistance exercises back to back with little or no rest between exercises has been shown to be particularly effective[46]. Exercise sessions that combine cardio and strength exercises show favorable changes in both strength and cardiovascular fitness[111, 126]. If you hate cardio, but love to lift try:

- Total body conditioning classes;
- boot camp classes;
- group strength classes;
- strength exercises done back to back with cardio exercise in short 1:00 - 3:00 minute bouts.

Classes have been a popular mode of cardiovascular exercise for decades. The group interaction and fun environment has helped many gym members become regular exercisers. However, even in a class format you need to progress your exercise continually . Here are some ideas for increasing your cardiovascular fitness in a class format:

- In classes that use weights or bands simply increase the resistance.
- Many step classes dictate tempo, however, you could raise your step. A study examining step height versus tempo reported an increase in step height as being more difficult[22].
- Try a different class. Any change in your program is likely to create a need for adaptations, and not all classes provide the same level of intensity. One study found cardio-kickboxing to be more intense than aerobic dance[4].
- Speak to your instructor about exercise progressions. Classes are aimed at the masses, not necessarily at the advanced member. Most instructors will have ideas on how to progress some of the exercises or steps.

Aqua running is a fun and challenging idea for cardio. Studies show significant benefit especially for older adults who benefit from the reduced stress on joints[33, 88].

Try a new machine. With more and more cardio machines entering the club every year there is plenty of opportunity to try something new. Challenge yourself.

Increase the intensity on the piece of cardio equipment you currently use. Most machines offer various adjustments, in speed, resistance, incline, stride frequency, or program. Set a goal, and work diligently to get there.

Sports are often a fun and challenging way to step up your cardio. A study showed individuals were better motivated to participate in sports and activities perceived to be fun, when compared to structured exercise programs[68, 140-141]. Various sports have been shown to have benefits for improving cardiovascular fitness. Studies have examined everything from competitive dance, to boxing, ice hockey, and even Tae Kwon Do[72, 119, 127, 139].

Structured exercise programs: Personal training, educational workshops, and text written by qualified fitness professionals may be the next step for you. A structured exercise program designed for your needs may lead to the best performance of your life, and better health too. It is important to change your program continually, and modify the intensity of your program as your body adapts. Many measures of cardiovascular performance-- including increased aerobic capacity, a higher VO2MAX, increased heart rate reserve, and quicker recovery from exercise -- are correlated with a significant decrease in the risk of cardiovascular disease[15, 25, 32, 42, 110]. All can be easily attained with a structured aerobic program, or regular participation in sport.

If your goal is weight loss you can find a listing of the caloric expenditure of various activities, including sports, at MyPyramid. gov. (Not to be confused with a fake site set up as MyPyramid.org.)

Myth #56: *Cardio should be done at a certain time.*
What You Should Know: Do cardio whenever you can, but prioritize and order your training according to your goal.

Cardiovascular training done after resistance training was perceived as harder[105]. If cardiovascular performance is your priority it is suggested that you start with cardiovascular activity and finish with resistance training, or perform resistance training on alternate days. If resistance training is your priority do cardio at the end of your workout. Cardiovascular activity may adversely affect your resistance training for up to 8 hours post training[143]. When you exercise is a matter of personal preference and has no bearing on the amount of calories or fat you burn.

Myth #57: *The calorie counters on cardio equipment are accurate.*
What You Should Know: They're close, but likely overestimate the amount of calories you burn.

Assuming that most equipment uses the established metabolic equations set forth by the ACSM (admittedly, a pretty large assumption) it is safe to say they are close, but studies have shown that these equations have a tendency to overestimate[109, 115]. At the very least the calorie counters on equipment are an excellent way to track your progress.

Frequency, intensity, and duration may be similar and can be expressed as total caloric expenditure[13]. Often variables within a program can be adjusted in a variety of ways to elicit similar results. For example:

- You may decide to take a ten minute walk before work, at lunch, and again when you get home to reach your goal of 30 minutes a day. In doing so you have increased the frequency of activity and decreased the duration, but you burned the same amount of calories.
- You may decide that jogging for 20 minutes is more enjoyable than walking for 40 minutes, the caloric burn is similar.
- You may hate to jog and actually prefer longer lower intensity walks, double the duration and you could burn the same number of calories.

Myth #58: *Sweating is good indicator of intensity, and is a great way to lose weight*
What You Should Know: Sweat is not a reliable indicator of intensity or fat loss.

Running outside on a hot day will make you sweat, but that is hardly a sign that you are working hard or shedding pounds. The weight you lose during sweating is water weight. The weight will return as soon as you ingest enough fluid to offset the fluid lost during activity. In a nutshell, you're losing weight, but the wrong kind, and it is not long-lasting.

Adding insult to injury, your body does not perform as well in the heat. Performing your cardiovascular activity outside during a hot day may cause dehydration, heat illness (such as heat stroke), and cardiovascular drift (an increase in heart rate not associated with an increase in activity). Although drinking plenty of fluids may help decrease risks, it will likely do little to offset fluid lost during sweating, or prevent a reduction in your performance[135-137]. It is not absurd to extend the results from these studies to include excessive body heat caused by exercising in rubber suits, and/or excessive clothing.

Further, in a study on collegiate runners comparing the indoor/winter season and the outdoor/summer season there was very little change in running economy, body temperature, and sweat rate after 17.5 weeks of training in the outdoor environment suggesting that the body has very little ability to adapt to a hot environment[16].

The Power of the Mind:

Verbal encouragement, training with a partner, and listening to your favorite tunes may improve your performance. These additions to your training actually have an effect on your physiology! Research suggests that verbal encouragement decreases rate of perceived exertion[14]. Social support increased enjoyment and actually reduced heart rate during exercise when compared to cardio at the same work load without social support[51]. Listening to self-selected music lowered heart rate, lowered systolic blood pressure; subjects had increased lactate at fatigue (possibly suggesting more resilience to lactic acid accumulation), had more favorable hormone response, and increased their time to exhaustion[41]. Adding a partner or music player may be just what you need to reach your goal.

The Gender Gap and Cardiovascular Performance:

We all know there is a small but significant difference in athletic abilities between men and women. Unfortunately it would seem that women have some physiological cards stacked against them.

How women differ:

- A propensity towards a higher body fat percentage, in essence, more non-working weight to carry around
- A smaller heart per body size requiring a higher heart rate at the same relative intensity
- Lower stroke volume (The heart does not pump as much blood with each beat)
- Less oxygen carrying red blood cells requiring a larger cardiac output for the same workload[18, 43, 52]

On the plus side men and women respond similarly to exercise[28, 52]. I have met many fit females who could beat the pants off their male counterparts. Take Joy Brookbush who performed better than many of her male peers on the Las Vegas Fire & Rescue physical examination to earn a spot with the LVFR fighting fires and saving lives. Congratulations Sis'.

How Your Body Adapts to Cardiovascular Exercise:

Excess weight and a sedentary lifestyle is a slow but sure killer. As your body fat slowly increases so do your chances of premature death. As our society becomes more technologically advanced and the prevalence of desk jobs increases, the "Coach Potato Bug" is biting more and more people every day.

Frightening Fact: Almost two-thirds of the adult population in the U.S. is overweight. A third of the population is not only overweight, but falls into the category of obese (NHANES 2005). Obesity has become the second leading cause of preventable death in this country, falling just behind smoking. As the percentage of new smokers continues to decline and our nation continues to get fatter, obesity is expected to become the number one cause of preventable death.

For your health: Don't get bitten by the couch potato bug

- Carrying excess body fat, leading a sedentary lifestyle and low cardiovascular fitness increase your risk for cardiovascular disease[26, 34, 39, 47, 49, 57, 67, 70]. All people, regardless of age, race, cultural background, education, or gender have been affected[39, 47-49, 56, 57, 67, 84, 87, 116, 129, 133]. Although you may read a report that older, African-American men are at the highest risk, a young Chinese girl on the other side of the globe is not free from risk. Globalization will assuredly pass the couch-potato bug to our neighbors if we do not change our habits.

The solution to this epidemic is simple: EXERCISE

- Any form of exercise - recreational activities, such as gardening, housework, walking, or more vigorous activities such as structured exercise programs and sports will decrease your risk of cardiovascular disease[3, 32, 39, 53, 56-57, 69, 103, 113, 129, 130].

The best time to start is NOW

- Studies show that individuals of all ages can improve their performance and reduce their risk of disease with a cardio program[35, 57, 84, 95, 134].

All exercise, regardless of the duration and/or intensity, must utilize the cardio-respiratory system to either sustain an activity and/or recuperate from it[27]. Specifically, if you wish to do anything for 90 seconds or more, or wish to increase the intensity of an activity that lasts longer than 3 minutes, cardiovascular training will likely have a direct effect on your performance.

Physiological Adaptations to Cardiovascular Exercise[18, 27, 52, 92, 98]

Respiratory system:
- Enhanced oxygen exchange in the lungs
- Improved blood flow throughout the lungs
- Decreased sub-maximal respiratory rate
- Decreased sub-maximal pulmonary ventilation

Cardiovascular System:
- Increased Cardio output
- Decreased heart rate at sub maximal workloads, decreasing the heart's need for oxygen
- Increase in stroke volume, first without changes in ventricle wall thickness, only changing end-diastolic volume
- Increased left ventricle wall thickness (92)
- Increased blood volume, red blood cell number and hemoglobin concentration
- Enhanced blood flow to skeletal muscle
- Decreased Exercise Blood Pressure (98)
- Positive adaptations in peripheral vascular system (larger conduit, and resistance vessel structures) (Naylor)
- Improved thermoregulation

Musculoskeletal system:
- Increased mitochondrial size and density. Increased mitochondria increases aerobic ATP production; therefore, reducing lactic acid production and the onset of fatigue
- Increased oxidative enzyme concentrations
- Increased myoglobin concentrations
- Increased capillarization in muscle bed (capillary to muscle fiber ratio)

- Increased arteriovenous oxygen difference
- Endurance training increases the number of mitochondria and capillaries in muscle, causing all fibers to become more oxidative, the effect is manifested in the increase of type IIa fiber and a decrease in type IIb
- Increased mitochondria increases aerobic ATP production; therefore, reducing lactic acid production and the onset of fatigue

Metabolic System:
- Increased Utilization of fat for fuel during activity and rest
- Increased Glycogen Storage

Integrated System Improvements: (Improvements in performance via increased production from more than one system and or the improved synergy between systems)
- Increased speed of oxygen transport kinetics
- Increased VO2Max
- Increased Lactic Acid Threshold
- Reduced time to reach steady state, therefore reducing oxygen debt and reliance on anaerobic ATP production
- Improved Exercise Economy (ex. Increased neuromuscular control, improving efficiency of the kinetic chain)
- Significant Improvements in recovery from oxygen debt and return to resting heart rate

Chapter 8:
Stretching Stuff

Flexibility may be the most neglected aspect of a comprehensive exercise routines. Many individuals will make time for cardio, resistance training, working the muscles of the mid section, but few spend time on a flexibility program. Then again, how could anyone spend time on an aspect of fitness that has been left so vague, is full of contradicting information, and is seldom explained in much detail? I have yet to see a popular magazine list the benefits of a flexibility program or give straight forward, practical advice, based on current research.

Myth #59: *I don't have time to stretch.*
What You Should Know: Stretching is one of the most accessible forms of exercise and results can be seen with just a couple of well executed stretches.

Better results may be seen if you do several 30-90 second repetitions per stretch (steps 3-5 of the instructions above), stretch every tight muscle, and utilize a variety of techniques, but it is not necessary to see results.

- One 30-90 second stretch per muscle will suffice. In a study measuring improvements during a static stretch held for 2:00 minutes and repeated several times, most of the increase in flexibility was seen within the first 30 seconds of the stretch and by the second repetition[54].

- Stretch for a few minutes at the end of each exercise session. Research on flexibility has compared frequencies ranging from just two sessions per week to twice daily[23, 27, 57, 89, 117, 119, 125]. Two times per week seems to be the minimum number of sessions to continue making gains, but you are not likely to see any benefit from stretching more than twice a day[3, 8, 30].
- Create a home stretching program. Stretching is not affected by watching the TV, reading the paper, or whether or not you performed the stretches in the gym, and the best part is you may not need any equipment. Optimally, stretch every day, whenever and wherever you can.
- Only stretch tight muscles. Choose a couple of tight muscles that would benefit from a good stretch. There is no need to stretch every muscle.

Benefits of Flexibility Training

- **May decrease instances of lower-back pain:** It is estimated that 80% of the adult population has suffered from, or is currently suffering from lower-back pain[29]. A lack of flexibility or range-of-motion in the hips and lower back may be a prognostic indicator of low back pain[67]. Most often rehabilitation for low back pain includes a stretching program to address any such issues.
- **Decrease chances of age related losses in flexibility:** Studies show an age-related loss in flexibility which could lead to injury and/or loss of function as we age[6, 7, 29, 30, 40, 122].
- **Stretching burns calories[106]:** Stretching may not be as effective as cardio, or even resistance training at melting away that fat, but all the calories you burn add up at the end of the day. You can increase your flexibility and burn calories, while watching your favorite TV program.
- **Increases blood flow to muscles stretched[58]:** Stretching may be useful in reducing cramping associated with ischemia (insufficient blood flow to a muscle).

146

- **Move Better:** A comprehensive flexibility program may decrease restrictions caused by muscular tightness. This will make movement easier and improve the efficiency of your muscular system[29, 30].
- **Recovery from orthopedic injury:** Several research studies have noted a decrease in flexibility program with the occurrence of pain and injury[20, 59, 64]. Studies have noted the importance of a comprehensive flexibility program when recovering from injury[20, 64, 87, 116]. However, I urge you to consult an orthopedic physician and/or a physical therapist for detailed instruction in incidence of injury or pain.
- **Decrease post exercise soreness:** Stretching and yoga have been shown to decrease the occurrence of post exercise soreness[8, 17].
- **Stretching helps reduce stress:** In a study examining stress reduction methods in Brazilian pre-university students, stretching significantly reduced symptoms[134].
- **Stretching post exercise may increase your performance in your next work-out:** In one study, those individuals who stretched after a workout intense enough to induce soreness performed better during an exercise session 48 hours later than those who did not[136].

Rules for Stretching:

Rule# 1: A muscle will adaptively shorten if it remains in a shortened position for too long, or if a muscle is used repetitively through a limited range of motion.

- If you slouch, your shoulders round forward, you hunch over a desk all day, or you sleep on your side, you may cause your chest muscles to shorten and become tight. If your pecs (the large muscles on your chest) become tight it could cause you soreness in your shoulders, a decrease in strength, and eventual injury.

- The "hip-flexors", a group of muscles crossing the front of the hip, have a tendency to become tight. These muscles are shortened when you sit behind a desk, in your car, on the couch, or sleep in a fetal position. These muscles will eventually adapt to this shortened position and could lead to pain in your low back and hips. It may also affect the normal function of other hip muscles like your gluteus maximus - your tush. Your "glutes" are very important to everyday movements such as walking, running, jumping, or getting out of a chair. But let's talk vanity for a moment. If this muscle stops functioning well, it could lead to the dreaded "droopy glute syndrome." You may be able to increase muscle tone in your glutes by performing a simple hip flexor stretch, and doing a few squats to get your glutes back in the mix.

- Many individuals come home complaining that their neck and trapezius muscles are tight and sore. Usually this is attributed to stress, but this may be another case of tightness. When you look at your computer screen at work, watch the road while driving, or stare at the TV while in bed, you may notice that your head is in a forward position and your trapezius and other muscles of your neck will adaptively become tight and short. If your head protrudes forward when you stand, you may have what was once referred to as "computer geek posture." Not limited to geeks anymore, this is very common in our technologically-advanced society. Holding your head in this position causes a lot of the muscles in your neck and the muscles above your shoulders to become very tight and possibly sore.

- Many women spend their day in high-heel shoes. In high-heel shoes, your calves are in a shortened or tight position and are only able to move through a shortened range of motion when you walk. The body will adapt, and your calves will become tight. This is most evident when a person gets home and is sore in the back of their lower legs, or experiences cramping in the lower leg. A simple calf stretch, and wearing flat shoes may alleviate this problem.

148

Rule# 2: Stretching tight muscles helps us maintain balance between muscle groups that would otherwise be disrupted by our daily activity.

I have met many gifted athletes, body-builders, fitness models, and recreationally active individuals who feel that their level of flexibility and mobility will have little impact on their performance.

What they don't know is that stretching will reduce restriction, and improve the efficiency of their muscular system[29, 30]. A good flexibility program can help every individual do what they do better. All systems in the body must perform in harmony to create optimal movement[29, 30]. One component of this harmonious relationship is the relative length of muscles surrounding a joint, termed length/tension relationship. Every muscle has an optimal length in which it can produce the most force. If a muscle becomes tight and short it not only decreases its ability to produce force, but it will likely affect the relative length of all the muscles crossing that joint. If all the muscles crossing that joint are no longer at their optimal length/tension then no muscle crossing that joint will be able to work to its potential, leaving that joint unable to produce optimal force.

Interesting Tidbit: One study found that most middle aged and older women fell well below standard norms for flexibility[19].

Examples of Stretching Leading to Improved Performance:

- Your pectoralis major (the large muscle in your chest) controls movement of the shoulder joint. This muscle has a tendency to become tight. Factors contributing to this tightness may include poor posture, hunching over a desk all day, overuse, or an imbalance caused by chest work without an equal amount of upper back work. If you have tightness in your chest, not only will it affect your chest movements in exercises   like bench press, flys, and machine press, but it will also affect any movements that requires movement of the shoulder joint. This includes all of your back work, your shoulder work, and to a lesser degree your arm work. Your entire upper body programming can be affected by tightness that started with just one muscle. This is a common postural distortion that may be improved upon by stretching your chest.

- A client of mine walked into the gym and wanted to improve his golf game. After a few quick assessments, I realized he had limited flexibility in his hips -- The likely cause of which was sitting behind a desk all day. Every time he swings his golf club and tries to turn through his hips, he has to overcome that restriction. This may cause him to lose some of the force that could be directed towards the ball. By simply teaching him a few hip stretches he could do at the gym or at home I gave him a routine that could be done daily. Within a couple of weeks he dramatically improved his hip flexibility, and added 15 yards to his drive.

- I was walking through the gym and noticed a rather "buff" gentleman doing overhead shoulder press with dumbbells. His form was awful. Every time he pressed the weight up, he had to arch his back and press his head back into the bench. Arching during a shoulder press is a common symptom of tightness in the latissimus dorsi. These are the large muscles in your back responsible for pulling your arms back down to your sides. This individual was trying to push up, but he was tight in the muscles that pull down. His tight lats caused a restriction that he had to overcome to push the weight up. I approached him and asked, "Do you have two minutes?" He gave me just enough time to show him a stretch for his tight lats, and when he returned to his overhead press, not only did he lift the weight with better form, but he was able to lift 10 more pounds.

How should I stretch?

Static stretching is the best option for most individuals based on effectiveness, the ability to perform the technique on yourself, and the relative ease of learning the techniques. Most studies comparing static stretching to other methods find it to be the most effective method for improving flexibility long term. The only method found to be more effective than static stretching (in a few, but not all studies) is PNF (proprio-neural facilitation) stretching, but this stretching technique requires the assistance of a certified professional[39, 48, 78]. Other stretching techniques offer unique benefits, but are likely best learned under the supervision of a certified, and/or licensed professional. (See "A Brief on Other Techniques" below.)

Stretching Instructions:

1. Elongate the muscle to a point of mild tension or discomfort and hold that position quietly and calmly. Pay close attention to your form. You should feel the stretch in the desired area.
2. Hold the stretch for 30 to 90 seconds until you feel a release, or reduction in discomfort. You should notice that the release or reduction in discomfort is accompanied by a small increase in your flexibility.
3. Elongate the muscle again until you reach a new point of mild discomfort or tension.
4. Hold this position for 30 to 90 seconds until you feel a release, a reduction in pain, or note an increase in your range of motion.
5. Again elongate the muscle to a point of mild discomfort, and hold this last position for 30 to 90 seconds until there is a feeling of release, or reduction in discomfort.

Myth #60: *Holding stretches for 5-10 seconds is enough to increase my flexibility.*
What You Should Know: 30 seconds or more per stretch is necessary for long-term improvements.

It is unlikely that stretches held for less than 30 seconds will create any long term change in your flexibility. In most studies holding a stretch for 30 seconds or more increased flexibility[23, 27, 48, 54, 57, 68, 86, 93, 101, 117, 119, 121, 125]. Conversely, studies holding a stretch for less than 30 seconds did not consistently result in increased flexibility[28, 56, 71-73, 77, 103, 125, 133].

Myth #61: *Stretching is most effective when you pull as hard as you can, and really make it hurt.*
What You Should Know: Not necessary and not effective.

Stretches should be held at a point of mild discomfort, and held at this point until the discomfort disappears. You should get a feeling of release. Stretching is about relaxation. The harder you pull on a muscle, the harder it will pull back. If you stretch so hard that your body feels it is in danger of injury, you are unlikely to ever get the muscle to relax and lengthen. A study examining stretch tolerance found that surpassing an individual's tolerance was not more effective in increasing flexibility[23].

Myth #62 *Lifting will mess up my flexibility.*
What You Should Know: Lifting will not blunt the effects of a flexibility program[112].

Certain types of training may exacerbate tightness, as athletes often exhibit flexibility below the norm. However, this should not deter any individual from lifting or stretching. Both types of exercise are incredibly beneficial and complement each other well. In a study comparing stretching alone versus stretching and resistance training, both groups made identical gains[112].

When Should I Stretch?

Stretch whenever you can -- at the end of your work-out, when you wake-up in the morning, or in the evening while you're watching

TV. Avoid stretching just before you lift, unless recommended by a health/wellness professional. The immediate effects of static stretching may actually inhibit a muscles ability to perform. Studies have recently suggested that static stretching and PNF stretching reduce force output of the affected musculature, especially when performing activities that require maximal amounts of speed, strength , or endurance[10, 18, 26, 35-36, 38, 45, 47, 51, 60, 72-73, 76, 93, 101, 103-105, 108, 110, 115, 121, 135, 142-143]. That is to say that the muscles involved in the stretch will not be as strong immediately following the stretch, and may be affected for up to two hours[115]. Static stretching is a process that relies on a muscles ability to relax (autogenic inhibition), so that a new length may be reached. If you relax a muscle and then ask it to move, the muscle may be unable to act in optimal fashion. Try to remember a time that you were startled out of a nap or forced to move quickly upon first waking. You probably felt a little clumsy and unable to respond as effectively. It takes time for you to wake up and function at full capacity, just as it may take time and a good warm-up to perform optimally after stretching. The simplest strategy is to start your program with a low to moderate intensity warm-up (i.e. the treadmill or stair-master) and finish your routine with a good stretching routine.

Note: Static stretching before your work-out is not always a negative. Postural dysfunction and injury may create a need for specific stretching techniques before activity to improve performance and reduce the risk of further injury. A health/fitness professional can help you develop a stretching routine specific to these issues.

Myth #63: *If you can touch your toes, you're flexible.*
What You Should Know: That's a good start, but you're not done.

The ability to touch your toes with your legs straight is a good start, but this only measures flexibility through a few joints, and in one direction. There is no one test, movement, or exercise that will determine your flexibility. All joints need to have a certain ROM in multiple directions to ensure proper joint function. This allows joints to move freely without pain, and reduces the risk of injury.

If a muscle becomes tight/overactive, or too long/under active it can lead to a change in body mechanics. If force is not distributed optimally throughout joints certain tissues will become over stressed. Those tissues that have become over stressed may break down over time causing pain. This often causes a viscous cycle of tightness, injury, pain, more tightness, etc. Flexibility may decrease with the occurrence of pain and injury[20, 59, 64].

Every time I walk in the gym I see individuals stretching what feels good, or doing the stretches they have always done. Often the muscles we have always stretched are no longer the muscles that are tight, and continuing to stretch these muscles is not recommended. It is doubtful that any further gains will be made, and if gains are made this could lead to hyper-mobility. Hyper-mobility is just as detrimental as a lack of flexibility. For example, most individuals have short/tight hip-flexors (see hip flexor stretch below), and hamstrings that have been pulled into a lengthened position. However, more people stretch their hamstrings creating the potential for hyper-mobility.

Only stretch muscles that are short and tight. Below are several tests you can perform at home to determine your flexibility issues and a couple of recommended stretches for each restriction.

Practical Self-Assessment:

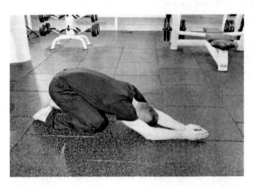

Child's Pose: Can you get on your knees, sit back on your heels, lie down forward so that your belly is resting on your legs, and reach your arms straight out above your head? You should be able to bring your head within a couple inches of the floor and still keep your arms fully extended over your head. If you cannot perform this test, stretch your lats and chest (described below).

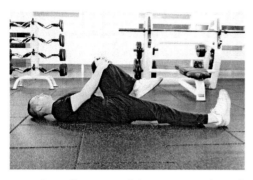

Modified Thomas Test: Lying on your back with one leg flat against the ground, can you bring the opposite leg close to your chest without the leg on the floor moving? If the leg on the ground leaves the floor, your knee bends, or your foot turns out you need to stretch your hip-flexors, adductors, and piriformis (described below).

Squat test: Starting with your feet parallel to each other (2nd toe pointing forward) and hip-width apart perform 5 to 10 squats without letting your heels leave the floor. If you do not know how to squat - lightly touch your butt on a chair as if you were going to sit down, but before you sit down stand right back up. Do this several times. If you finish and notice that your heels have caved inward or your feet point out it is likely that your calves and other lower body musculature have become tight. Stretch your calves, hip flexors, and adductors (described below).

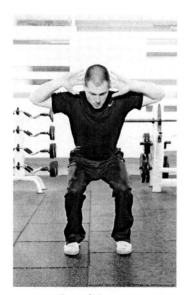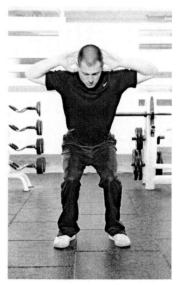

Good Squat   Bad Squat

The muscles assessed in the tests above are termed "tonic," which means they have a propensity to become tight, short, and/or overactive[29, 30]. If you cannot perform one of the tasks in the graph above, start each day or exercise routine with the stretches recommended for that task. If you feel pain through any of these assessments it may be necessary for you to consult a qualified fitness professional, physical therapist, or orthopedic physician.

If you find the above tests to be confusing, below is a list (in order of priority) of muscles that have a propensity to become tight, and simple stretches for each muscle.

1. Calves
2. Hip Flexors
3. Latissimus Dorsi
4. Chest
5. Piriformis
6. Adductor

Calve Stretch (Arrows indicate where you should feel the stretch):

1. Find a wall or solid object to lean against.
2. Take a large step back with the leg you wish to stretch.
3. Ensure that both feet are pointing straight ahead.
4. With your back leg - squeeze your glutes (butt muscles) and quads (lock your knee), and press your heel into the floor.
   - At this point you may feel a mild stretch. If you do – hold the position.
   - If you do not feel a stretch - slide your hips forward, keeping your heel on the ground, until you feel a light stretch.
5. Hold the position for at least 30 seconds – ideally, hold that position until you feel a release or significant reduction in discomfort.

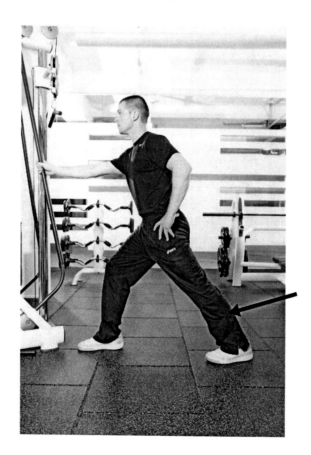

Hip Flexor Stretch (Arrows indicate where you should feel the stretch)**:**

1. Find a wall or solid object to use for support.
2. Assume a kneeling position (the shin of your front leg should be perpendicular to the floor).
3. Ensure that your hips, knees, and feet are in alignment.
4. Draw your belly button toward your spine and "get tall."
5. Tuck your tail bone underneath you (posterior pelvic tilt) and squeeze your glutes.
6. Shift your hips forward until you feel a stretch in the front of your hip (of the back leg).
7. Hold the position for at least 30 seconds – ideally, hold that position until you feel a release or significant reduction in discomfort.

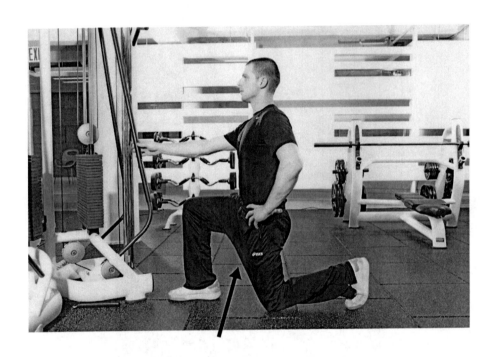

Latissimus Dorsi Stretch a.k.a. Child's Pose (Arrows indicate where you should feel the stretch)**:**

1. Get down on both knees and sit back on your heels.
2. Lay forward so that your belly is now resting on your legs.
3. Reach your arms straight out above your head with thumbs pointing up.
4. Allow gravity to pull your head and torso toward the floor.
5. As you sink deeper toward the floor you should notice a significant stretch underneath your arms and between your shoulder blades.
6. Hold that position for at least 30 seconds – ideally, hold that position until you feel a release or significant reduction in discomfort.

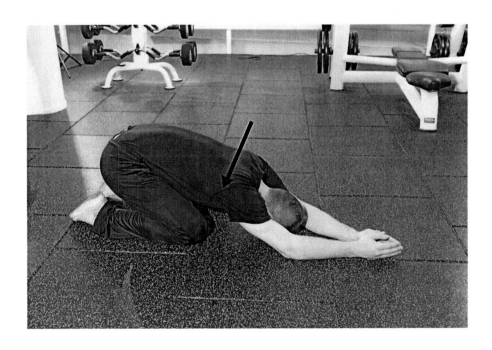

Chest Stretch (Arrows indicate where you should feel the stretch)**:**

1. Find a wall or solid object.
2. Extend your arm behind the object, reaching higher than shoulder level (your elbow should remain above your shoulder for the duration of the stretch).
3. Get as tall as you can, draw your belly button toward your spine and squeeze your glutes.
4. Lean forward so the object is pulling your arm up, back, and away from your body.
5. Keep going until you feel a mild stretch.
6. Hold that position for at least 30 seconds – ideally, hold that position until you feel a release or significant reduction in discomfort.

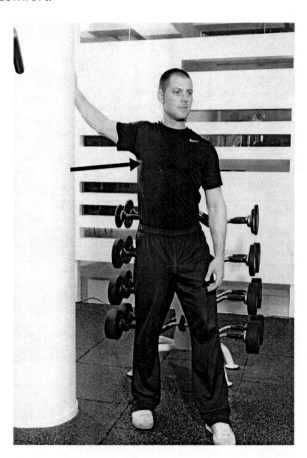

Adductors (Arrows indicate where you should feel the stretch)**:**

1. Take a wide stance (about double hip width).
2. Take a small step back with the leg you want to stretch (the toe of your back leg should line up with the heel of your front leg).
3. Tuck your tailbone underneath you (posterior pelvic tilt) and squeeze your glutes.
4. Shift your hips toward your front leg until you feel a stretch.
5. Use your hand to depress and stabilize the hip your stretching.
6. Hold that position for at least 30 seconds – ideally, hold that position until you feel a release or significant reduction in discomfort.

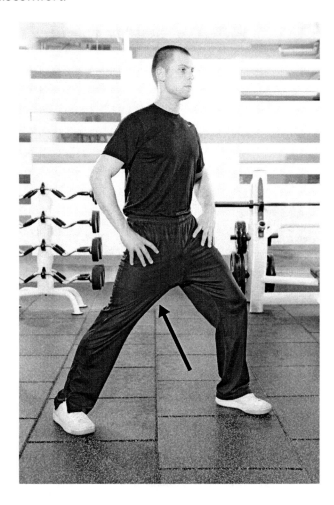

Piriformis (Arrows indicate where you should feel the stretch)**:**

1. Lay on your back with your backside close to a wall or solid object.
2. Place one foot up on the wall (your hip and knee should form 90° angles).
3. Cross your opposite leg and rest your ankle on your knee.
4. Use your hands to press the "crossed" knee away from you.
5. You should feel a stretch in the back or your hip (of the leg that is crossed).
6. Hold that position for at least 30 seconds – ideally, hold that position until you feel a release or significant reduction in discomfort.

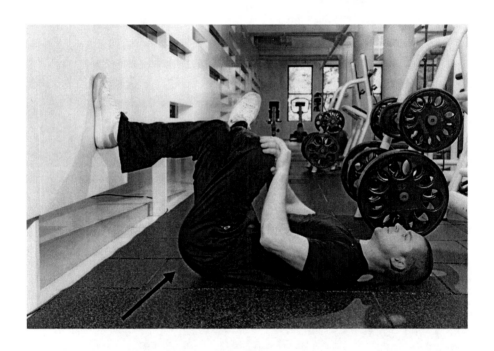

Note: Some individuals may have other needs, may not be tight in the muscles listed, or may need different stretching techniques to attain optimal results. If you find the following to be ineffective, please consult a health/fitness professional.

Stretching and Injury Prevention

If you played an organized sport, had gym in school, or read popular fitness magazines you knew that you had to stretch before you started activity. It was part of our warm-up to prevent muscle tears, pulls, and other such injuries. I know many individuals who took that thought one step further, believing that the more flexibility they had, the better off they were. Well unfortunately, it just doesn't work that way.

Current research has found no relationship between pre-activity stretching and a reduction in the incidence of injury[111, 114, 129]. In fact, studies have shown pre-activity static stretching may actually reduce a muscles ability to produce force[10, 18, 26, 35-36, 38, 45, 47, 60, 72-73, 76, 93, 101, 103-105, 108, 110, 115, 121, 135, 142-143]. That is not to say that stretching is bad for you. Optimal levels of flexibility will enhance your performance and may reduce the risk of injury; however, optimal flexibility is a long term adaptation that may takes several sessions to achieve. One stretching session before you work-out will not solve your problem.

Chronic stretching has been shown to increase performance[102, 136]. But, it is also important to note that too flexible may be a hindrance. Many studies have shown increased performance with runners who are actually tighter in their hips and ankles[36, 69, 109]. Optimal flexibility does not mean as flexible as possible, it means just the right amount of flexibility. Being too flexible, termed "hyper-mobility" may be just as dangerous as being too tight.

At the end of each exercise session, we should do our best to stretch muscles that are short and tight, not just the muscles and stretches that feel good. Identifying those muscles that are short and tight and building your flexibility program around those stretches will ensure you don't "overstretch" already loose muscles.

Myth # 64: *You have to warm-up before you stretch.*
What You Should Know: A warm-up has no effect on the long-term benefits made from a stretching program.

Warm-Up activities have no effect on the gains you will make from a stretching program; however, a warm-up may enhance your flexibility for a short time immediately following the warm-up[15, 50, 55, 113, 137].

A Brief on Other Techniques:

There are various other methods of stretching. Each technique has its own unique purpose and set of parameters. Due to the complex nature of these other techniques it is suggested that the reader consult a healthcare professional for further advice. Below I have summarized some of these techniques so that you, the reader, are aware of all of your options as you progress through your fitness routine.

1. Active Stretching:

Lie on your back and grab one leg behind your knee with both hands. Contract your thigh muscles to extend your knee until you feel a stretch in your hamstring, hold and repeat. This is active stretching. Active stretching is a term used to describe a stretch that involves an active contraction of the opposing musculature (the quads in the example above) to lengthen a muscle (the hamstrings in the example above) to its end range. Generally these stretches are held for two to five seconds and repeated six to 10 times[30, 81]. One of the benefits associated with this form of stretching is an increase in strength and control through the new range of motion acquired with this technique.

2. Dynamic Stretching:

Dynamic Stretching is a wonderful addition to your warm-up routine. Dynamic stretching uses the force produced by muscles and the body's momentum to take a joint through a full available range of motion[29, 30]. This technique utilizes dynamic activities such as leg swings, lunges, butt-kicks, and axe chops, to stretch muscles at a tempo that is more activity specific. With these stretches being done as fast as the individual can control, the risk of injury increases and it is suggested that a fitness professional be consulted when learning and growing accustomed to a dynamic flexibility program. This stretching technique may be the best method for warming-up in the intermediate to advanced individual. Several studies have shown an increase in performance post dynamic stretching[47, 51, 140, 142].

3. PNF Stretching:

For the purpose of lengthening tight muscles and increasing mobility long term, research suggests that the most effective means of stretching is a technique termed PNF stretching[26, 39, 48, 49, 56, 78, 93, 101, 123]. PNF is short for Proprioceptive Neuromuscular Facilitation. There are three phases that should be repeated at least three times when using PNF stretching: relaxation in an elongated position, agonist contraction, and antagonist contraction. Research suggests that a muscle be elongated to the first resistance barrier, followed by at least a 6 - 10 second isometric contraction of the muscle being stretched[26, 33, 56, 93, 101, 121, 123], followed by a 10-30 sec contraction of the opposing musculature to bring you to the next tissue barrier[26, 49], followed by 15 to 30 seconds of rest in the new position[101], and then repeated[22, 32, 59, 101], optimally 3 times[123]. More research is desperately needed to update and further refine the length of each phase of this technique. This type of stretching is obviously complex, and for best results requires the assistance of an experienced certified professional, proficient in this technique[128].

4. Massage:

Two studies have shown an increase in flexibility with massage therapy[31, 74]. In both studies one muscle group was massaged for at least 10 minutes and both used deep tissue techniques. Only one of these studies in which massage was done three times a week for 10 weeks showed a long-term increase in flexibility[74].

5. Yoga, Pilates, and Tai Chi:

These modes of exercise focus on posture, control, and balance using large, slow movements through a complete range of motion. This is the likely reason they are effective for increasing flexibility and why they make great additions to your current exercise program[90]. Tai Chi in particular may have long lasting flexibility benefits. Long-time practitioners showed flexibility in the 90th percentile[65]. The poses in this beautiful art form require a significant amount of hip mobility and may be of great benefit to anyone looking to improve their lateral movement[80].

6. Foam Rolls:

Using foam rolls, sticks, or medicine balls for a technique called self-myofascial release shows promise as a means to reduce adhesions (knots), decrease hyper-activity in tight musculature and may be effective as a warm-up[29, 30, 98]. The research on these techniques, however, is limited and generally does not follow a set methodology. Often the protocol used varies from study to study.

Chapter 9:
Motivational Development

Myth # 65: *One day I'll be motivated to make a change.*
What You Should Know: Motivation is not ordained, it's developed.

Why is it that regardless of the risk, people will not commit to physical activity? They avoid exercise, make excuses, or get to the gym and just go through the motions. Our nation is getting fatter despite the availability of facilities and information on exercise. We need a shift in paradigm. And fast.

The allied health field is missing something. They are missing a piece of the puzzle that would make a healthy lifestyle a reality for everyone. It is not enough to simply try harder. The over-abundance of programs that are bigger, fancier versions of past programs, reminds me of the often quoted definition of insanity. "If you keep doing the same thing and expect a different result, you might be insane."

For most American's, a healthful lifestyle is a new behavior. The allied health field needs to redirect its focus from creating more activities to developing the habits and drives that would incorporate those activities. A great exercise routine, diet plan, or piece of equipment is only great if someone is motivated to use it. We must consider the amount of effort you are willing to expend, the sacrifices you're willing to make, the enthusiasm you have for living a healthy lifestyle, and the activities you enjoy. A healthy lifestyle requires more than an education in physical activity it requires an understanding of motivation; a plan that will ensure long-term commitment.

Myth # 66: *Joining your local gym will motivate you to start an exercise program.*
What You Should Know: Joining a gym provides you with a variety of tools, but motivation may not be one of them.

In times of a booming fitness industry and advancements in exercise science happening faster than ever before, it is hard to believe that less than 40% of Americans get the recommended levels of physical activity[8]. Only about 15% of Americans belong to a health club or related facility. The increase in the number of clubs has only created an industry where more health clubs fight for the same member. And with health clubs selling hundreds of memberships per year, you may be surprised to find that only 20% of their members use the gym on a regular basis, and many gyms lose 80% of their members each year. Those who are physically active possess these traits[12]:

1. A willingness to expend a moderately high amount of effort and intensity in pursuing their exercise
2. They enjoy exercise and they want to perform the activity for its own sake
3. When exercise was missed the individuals felt as though something was missing from their lives

Goals Are the Cornerstone of Motivation:

Many individuals go to the gym without a clear vision of what they want to accomplish. Usually they spend their time doing exercises that have little relevance to obtaining any particular goal, they are easily distracted, they talk more than they train, or work-out at an intensity that will not result in any change. They allow any immediately gratifying activity to take priority over their exercise program, and soon frustration and a lack of results diminishes motivation and participation in healthful activities stops. They may deem themselves as being lazy or unmotivated to exercise, but these would be wholly unfair judgments. How can you be lazy or unmotivated, if you are not trying to accomplish a goal? Here's an analogous scenario:

You get to work at your normal time, but your in-between projects so there is less to do than normal. No deadlines, no paperwork to do, a couple phone calls to make, but that's it. Your Boss walks in....

Boss: "Hurry up and get something done".

You: "Hurry up and get what done?"

Boss: I don't know. Just get busy.

You: "Yes, sir".

Boss: "Lazy Employee."

You start rumbling through paper work and counting paper clips.

Without clear-cut goals, you're not lazy, you're just "counting paper clips." You look busy, but how much are you really getting accomplished. Remember that motivation requires motive. Studies show, setting goals, both short-term and long-term, leads to a more effective plan of action, decreases the rate of dropout, and improves adherence[1, 22].

Goal Development:

A well developed goal must be: personal, attainable, create an appropriate level of challenge, and be positive, compelling, detailed, written, and time bound.

Personal: Every individual is different, and what works for one person may not work for another. Studies show that psychological differences, personality, gender, anatomical variables, exercise experience, body composition, body satisfaction, and whether an individual is overweight, or of normal weight all have a significant effect on motivation[10, 16, 26, 29, 31, 36, 37]. Try not to make someone else's goal your own; your goal must be personal or "intrinsic" in nature. For example, your doctor tells you that you need to work out, and supplies you with facts like exercise improves resting blood pressure, decreases your risk of atherosclerotic disease, increases glucose sensitivity, increases your bone density, and decreases your risk of all cause morbidity. These are important adaptations to exercise, but to a 30 year-old male five months before beach season, these goals may not be personally motivating. A 30 year-old who is working towards a better physique will be far more committed to an exercise program and still attain all of the benefits associated with exercise as a result.

Attainable: Everyone has individuals they admire, and achievements they revere, but we must maintain a realistic perception of what opportunities are available to each of us. I would love to have the athletic abilities of Lebron James, but a 6'3" clumsy kid does not pose the same threat on the court. By establishing a realistic goal, and remaining flexible as obstacles and limitations are faced, improvements will be made. Unattainable goals, a lack of flexibility and all-or-none thinking makes an individual more susceptible to the abstinence-violation effect, in which participants feel he or she has failed with any setback or missed goals[18].

Appropriate level of challenge: When establishing goals you must determine an appropriate level of challenge. Too much challenge relative to skill leads to anxiety and detachment, where as too little challenge leads to anxiety and boredom[9]. Optimal challenge is important in establishing true feelings of competence[9]. Try not to sell yourself short, but be careful to create a goal that does not surpass your level of commitment.

Positive: Using a technique called cognitive restructuring, change negative statements and thoughts into positive ones[22]. Example, you should restructure a goal like, "I *have* to lose weight, I'm so fat". Instead make the statement positive - "I really *want* (desire) a slim, sexy 28 inch waist and harder legs, by next summer; so I can fit into the size 6 suits in my closet. Negative feedback has been shown to have detrimental effects on performance, when compared to positive feedback and no feedback at all[3, 9, 34]. Research shows, negative feedback is undermining to feelings of competence, decreases intrinsic motivation (doing something because it is inherently enjoyable or interesting), and decreases autonomous behavior[3, 9, 34]. Further, negative feedback may promote "worry focus". A person who receives negative feedback may increase their attention on the problem, rather than staying focused on the solution[3].

Compelling: According to behavioral choice theory, engaging in physical activity usually involves choosing exercise over a concurrent and powerfully competing sedentary behavior[11]. If the goal is not compelling, most sedentary activities are going to seem more appealing than your exercise program. I love the following Tony Robbins quote which seems to embody this idea "You are not lazy, you simply have not found goals compelling enough to excite you."

Detailed: A vision of your ideal level of fitness will help give you leverage to change by noting a difference between where you are, and where you want to be. The clarity of your vision is extremely important. The more detailed your long-term goal, the more focus is created, the more leverage we have to create a change in behavior, and the better foundation we have to build a plan. If given the opportunity to build your dream house, would you simply tell a carpenter: "Build me a house"? The carpenter needs details, such as, where the house would be located, it's size, color, and what materials to use. To ensure that your vision of "ideal fitness" is achieved, you need to create a detailed path to follow. Your *vision* should not be weight loss. Instead, detail how much weight loss, by when, for what goal, and envision what effect that weight loss will have on your life.

Written: Whether long-term or short-term, you should write your goals down. In a study by psychologist Laura King, those individuals who wrote about their life goals grew more satisfied with their lives and more optimistic over time than those who wrote about a traumatic event, or about a neutral topic[4]. To write something down is to make a promise to yourself; a personal contract of sorts.

Time Bound: Setting a date is nothing more than procrastination prevention. Procrastination often leads to failure, or mediocre performance. Feelings of failure lead to self-blame, lowered self-esteem, guilt, perceived loss of control, increased probability of relapse, and possibility of giving up. However, each fulfilled action is an accomplishment. Each accomplishment increases an individual's sense of achievement, and achievement motivation has been found to be a strong predictor of continued success[35].

Myth # 67: *I have a goal and exercise equipment. I'm ready to go.*
What You Should Know: A goal is not action, it is intent to act. We still need a game plan.

Steps for Game Plan Development:

An inadequate plan, lack of commitment, and lack of revision can all contribute to relapse, or decrease in healthful activity[17].

1. **Create a long-term goal:** Use the guidelines above to create a well developed long-term goal.

2. **Create short-term/intermittent goals:** Short term goals help improve success rates by adding steps that are closer to an individual's current state[3]. For example, if 15 pounds of fat loss is the *vision*, then we may create a series of short term goals, for example, 5 pounds of fat loss per month.

3. **Create a list of behaviors that will lead to those goals:** If focus is placed on developing process or behavioral goals studies show an increased likelihood of success, and behavioral goals are easier to implement[22, 25]. Behavioral goals may include, frequency to the gym, activities that will be performed in and out of the gym, and how often. For example, if the short term goal is losing 5 pounds this month, behavioral goals may include committing to 30 minutes of cardio 4 days a week, 2 days of weight training per week, a promise not to eat garbage Monday through Friday, and joining a recreational volleyball league. Note: When creating process goals studies show sports and activities perceived to be fun, were more driven by intrinsic motivation, as opposed to structured exercise programs which were driven primarily by extrinsic regulation[20].

4. **Act on those behaviors:** This step is the most important. Develop a sense of urgency, and use this sense of urgency to accomplish a behavioral goal. Each accomplishment will increase your motivation. The increase in motivation will in turn lead to more activity, more accomplishments, and further

increase motivation. This could create a cycle of success that promotes self-worth and self-determination causing the anxiety and apathy for exercise to be replaced by feelings of competence and self-satisfaction. "You are more likely to act yourself into to feeling than feel yourself into action." – *Dr. Stephen R. Covey*

5. **Optimize:** Optimization is the practice of revision with efficiency in mind. When revising your game plan, do away with all-or-none thinking and keep the ego out of the way. Remaining flexible to change will help prevent relapse and allow you to take advantage of the variety of options available to you. Everybody faces unexpected obstacles and setbacks. This process will help to ensure that you do not reach the same obstacles time-and-time again.

- **Reflection → Forethought → Action → Repeat:**
  - **Reflection**: Look back and analyze previous methods, and identify barriers that lie between where you are now and where you want to be. Ask, "What did I do right, and what barriers did I face?"
  - **Forethought:** Once methods and results are tracked, work to eliminate barriers, and look forward to create a better path toward the vision. Ask, "What would I do differently?"
  - **Action:** Immediately, without haste, take action with the revised plan.
  - **Repeat:** After taking action, reflect once again on the method and result, and use forethought to plan the next action.

Some Pointers for Optimizing Your Exercise Program:

In general, diet and exercise do not create immediate change, and the delayed gratification will challenge your motivation. Relying on short term-goals at this point is a must. It is important to develop strategies to prevent sedentary behavior in advance. For example, decrease the amount of steps between leaving work and working-out by packing a gym bag and taking it with you to work. Increase the steps it takes to participate in a sedentary behavior, by taking the TV out of the bedroom. Instead put the TV in a room with space for your stretching, core routines, or in front of a piece of home exercise equipment.

Dr. Stephen Covey, author of *The Seven Habits of Highly Effective People* says it best. "Don't prioritize your schedule; schedule your priorities." Continually ask, "What is the most valuable use of my time right now?" List your long-term, short-term, and process goals developed in the previous step. List these goals in the order they should be accomplished, prioritize them, and set them to dates. This will preemptively solve time constraint problems that are bound to arise. At this point day timers, PDAs, and the worksheet below, may come in handy. Start by listing and prioritizing all the process goals that can be done daily. These are the activities that will develop into habits and make fitness a lifestyle. Continue with weekly goals, monthly goals, etc.

Be aware of the potential outcomes of not exercising, so the behavioral consequences of relapse are placed in proper perspective - minimize any tendency of interpreting a temporary relapse as total failure[22]. You must remain flexible. Everybody has off days, but consistant effort will create lifelong change. In a brief review of current research by O'Connor and Peutz, a positive relationship between physical activity and feeling energized was found[24].

Supporting Motivational Development:

The Self-Determination Theory, developed by Deci and Ryan, proposes the following "People will become more or less interested in activities as a function of the degree to which they experience need satisfaction while engaging in that activity[9]." The model is based on three fundamental needs.

Autonomy can be defined as the need to feel responsible for one's action.

Competence is a need to learn and be effective.

Relatedness is the need to feel support from another.

Strategies in support of fundamental needs and motivational development:

Autonomy:

- **Decisional Balance:** Do not allow someone else to dictate a routine to you. Do not copy a program out of a magazine. You need to play an active role in creating your progam. Making decisions leads to feeling responsible for the programs outcome. This may increase feelings of self-efficacy, self-determined behavior, and intrinsic motivation[9, 34]. Individuals who do not feel responsible for the outcome of a program may lose motivation, as intrinsic motivation is thwarted and replaced with controlled motivation[9].
- **Achievement Motivation:** Successful completion of activities will increase feelings of achievement, and therefore, achievement motivation. Achievement motivation can be defined as the feeling one gets after a win or the successful completion of a task. Achievement motivation has been shown to be a positive predictor of future success[35]. *"There is no joy like accomplishment."*

Competence:

- **Education:** An exercise program has a better chance of being followed if the individual understands the minimum amount of exercise that can lead to improvement, the exercise physiology behind the recommendation, and the physical and physiologic gains to be made from exercise[2]. Continued education should be part of a well designed game-plan. This may include lectures, articles, educational websites, books, or instruction from a fitness professional. Better education may also contribute to autonomy by providing you with the tools to make decisions when creating your exercise routine.

175

- **Repetition:** "Repetition is the mother of skill." Learning a new skill requires practice. It is unlikely you will be comfortable the first time. Practice new activities and skills and the result will be competence and comfort.

Relatedness:

- **Supportive Environment:** Create a support system for yourself. Find a work-out partner, look for support from family members, ask for emotional support from friends, or find a peer with similar goals. In a study by the Presidential Counsel of Physical Fitness and Sports, those individuals who received a greater number of counseling messages on fitness were more likely to become physically active than those receiving fewer messages[22].
- **Establish Role-Models:** Find positive role models or teachers to help you on your path. A smart man learns from his mistakes, a brilliant man learns from the mistakes of others. For example, in a study on novice weight lifters asked to select a weight that they thought was heavy enough, most chose weights that were unlikely to create changes in muscle strength or induce hypertrophy (growth)[14]. Choosing the appropriate weight for an exercise is easily demonstrated by a friend, teammate, work-out partner, or fitness professional you trust.

Myth # 68: *Reading this book will make your heart healthy, your muscles stronger, and fat melt-away like butter.*
What You Should Know: This book is a tool that you must put to use.

My motivation for writing this book was developed by accident. For years, I read popular fitness magazines, watched shows hosted by body builders, and took the labels on supplements as gospel. As I pursued my degrees and started reading books and research unbiased by the endorsement of supplements and marketing dollars, I realized that I had not been seeing the big picture.

More than ten years ago, the American College of Sports Medicine used the term "epidemic" to warn us about the serious health risks associated with our increasing levels of inactivity. And still, the epidemic continues with more than 60% of Americans overweight, and nearly one-third reaching clinical obesity (NHANES). Despite the Surgeon General's shift in paradigm, promoting that physical activity need not be strenuous to achieve health benefits, the obesity epidemic has been linked to the first expected decrease in life expectancy in recent history. Obesity related diseases include diabetes, high cholesterol, hypertension, heart disease, and orthopedic injury. These preventable diseases reduce the quality of life of millions of Americans. If that was not bad enough, the increase in healthcare costs associated with obesity related diseases could eclipse the economic growth of our country; undermining our economic stability, and create unprecedented levels of financial ruin for millions of Americans in as little as 10 years.

From these motivators and the need to help, I set my goals. I wanted to ensure that those starting an exercise program had the best information available (research/evidence based practice). Unfortunately, there seems to be a gap between the brightest minds in exercise science and the consumer. I wanted to ensure that fewer individuals are the victims of misinformation giving them the best chance for success. I wanted the information to be easy to read and use, and maybe enjoyable. Fitness doesn't have to be hard and painful and neither should reading about it. Combing through research, writing one chapter at a time, and editing several times I eventually finished this book. A heartfelt thank you to Sabila Khan, and my editor Rakia Clark for teaching a muscle-head/science-geek like me English composition, and for making me a decent writer.

The development of this book and the step toward your dreams are the same process. You need to know why you are getting fit. You need to create your game-plan, and you need to look for help when you need it. Heck, if this muscle-head can write a coherent book, a healthier meal can't be too hard to prepare.

In a way, this book is written backwards. Below I have created a worksheet that was built using the information in this chapter, and can be filled in with the information from previous chapters. When you have finished this worksheet, you will have a game-plan that makes your fitness goals more attainable.

With a little patience, persistence, and perseverance, you can attain most goals. Reading this book was a time commitment, done one page at a time, and it was huge step toward educating yourself. I hope that motivation, and drive for goal relevant education continues until you are looking back on where you were, as you stand where you want to be.

Motivational Development Worksheet:

Long Term Goal (6 Months or More)
Goals should be personal, attainable, create an appropriate level of challenge, be positive, compelling, detailed, written, and time bound.

_____

_____

Short Term Goals (3 Months or Less)
1.
2.
3.

Process or Behavioral Goals
Nutrition (Keep it simple, ex: less snacking, a smaller bowl for cereal or fewer alcoholic beverages)
1.
2.
3.

Recreational Activity (Ex: Sports you enjoy, walking on your lunch break, classes you enjoy)
1.
2.
3.

Cardio
Type:_____
Days Per Week:____
Minutes Per Session_____
Intensity_____ (ex. Heart Rate, Miles/Hour, Strides/Minute, Level, Distance)

Resistance Training:
Days Per Week____
Number of Exercises_____
Sets Per Exercise_____
Repetitions Per Set_____

Flexibility
Days Per Week_____
When: Morning   Lunch   Evening   Pre-Workout
Post-Workout
List Stretches: (Keep in mind that each stretch must be held for a minimum of 30 seconds per side)

1.
2.
3.
4.

Notes: (List strategies that will make healthful activities more accessible, keep track of how this program is working out, track progress, or just take notes of how you feel each day.)

Bibliography:
Section 1 – Chapters 1 & 2

1. Robert P. Ahmun, Richard J. Tong, and Paul N. Grimshaw. The Effects of Acute Creatine Supplementation on Multiple Sprint Cycling and Running Performance in Rugby Players. *J. Strength Cond. Res.* 19(1), 92-97, 2005, Copyright 2005 National Strength and Conditioning Association

2. American College of Sports Medicine. ACSM's Guidelines for Exercise Testing and Prescription, Sixth Edition; Senior Editor Barry A. Franklin, Associate Editor Mitchell H. Whaley and Edward T. Howley; Authors Gary J. Dalady.... [et. al.] Copyright 2001 American College of Sports Medicine

3. American College of Sports Medicine. Position Stand - Appropriate Intervention Strategies for Weight Loss and Prevention of Weight Regain for Adults. *Medicine & Science in Sports & Exercise* Copyright 2001 American College of Sports Medicine

4. American College of Sports Medicine. Position Stand - Exercise and Fluid Replacement. *Medicine and Science in Sports and Exercise: Volume 28(1) January 1996,* Copyright 2006 American College of Sports

5.   American College of Sports Medicine. Joint Position Statement - Nutrition and Athletic Performance. *Medicine &Science in Sports and Exercise* Copyright 2000 American College of Sports Medicine.

6.   American College of Sports Medicine. Roundtable - The Physiological and Health Effects of Oral Creatine Supplementation. *Medicine and Science in Sports and Exercise; 2000,* Copyright 2006 American College of Sports

7.   American College of Sports Medicine. Position Stand - The Recommended Quantity and Quality of Exercise for Developing and Maintaining Cardiorespiratory and Muscular Fitness, and Flexibility in Healthy Adults. *Medicine & Science in Sports & Exercise 30(6) June, 1998* Copyright 2006 American College of Sports Medicine

8.   Neva G. Avery, Jennifer L. Kaiser, Matthew J. Sharman, Timothy P. Scheett, Dawn M. Barnes, Ana L. Gomez, William J. Kraemer, and Jeff S. Volek. Effects of Vitamin E Supplementation on Recovery From Repeated Bouts of Resistance Exercise. *J. Strength Cond. Res.,* 2003, 17(4), 801-809, Copyright 2003 National Strength and Conditioning Association

9.   Thomas R. Baechle, Roger W. Earle. Essentials of Strength Training and Conditioning - 2nd Edition. Copyright 2000, 1994 National Strength and Condition Association

10. Bar-Or, Oded; Foreyt, John; Bouchard, Claude; Brownell, Kelly D.; Dietz, William H.; Ravussin, Eric; Salbe, Arline D.; Schwenger, Sandy; St. Jeor, Sachito; Torun Benjamin. Physical Activity, Genetic, and Nutritional Considerations in Childhood Weight Management. *Medicine and Science in Sports and Exercise: Volume 30(1) January 1998 pp. 2-10,* Copyright 2006 American College of Sports Medicine

11. Reinaldo A. Bassit, Leticia A. Sawada, Reury Frank P. Bacrau, Francisco Navarro, and Luis Fernando B. P. Costa Rosa. The Effect of BCAA Supplementation upon the Immune Response of Triathletes. *Medicine and Science in Sports and Exercise: Volume 32(7) 2000 pp 1214-1219*, Copyright 2006 American College of Sports Medicine

12. Louise J. Beaton, Damon A. Allan, Mark A. Tarnopolsky, Peter M. Tiidus, and Stuart M. Phillips. Contraction-Induced Muscle Damage is Unaffected by Vitamin E Supplementation. *Medicine and Science in Sports and Exercise: Volume 34(5) 2002 pp. 798-805*, Copyright 2006 American College of Sports Medicine

13. M. Daniel Becque, John D. Lochmann, and Donald R. Melrose. Effects of Oral Creatine Supplementation on Muscular Strength and Body Composition. *Medicine and Science in Sports and Exercise: Volume 32(3) 2000 pp 654-658*, Copyright 2006 American College of Sports Medicine

14. John M. Berardi and Tim N. Ziegenfuss. Effects of Ribose Supplementation on Repeated Sprint Performance in Men. *J. Strength Cond. Res.*, 2003, 17(1), 47-52, Copyright 2003 National Strength and Conditioning Association

15. Jason R. Berggren, Matthew W. Hulver, G. Lynis Dohm, and Joseph A. Houmard. Weight Loss and Exercise: Implications for Muscle Lipid Metabolism and Insulin Action. *Medicine and Science in Sports and Exercise: Volume 36(7) July 2004 pp 1191-1195*, Copyright 2006 American College of Sports Medicine

16. Craig J. Biwer, Randall L. Jensen, W. Daniel Schmidt, and Phillip B. Watts. The Effect of Creatine on Treadmill Running With High-Intensity Intervals. *J. Strength Cond. Res.* 17(3), 439-445, Copyright 2003 National Strength and Conditioning Association

17. Blair, Steven N.; Horton, Edward; Leon, Arthur S.; Lee, I-Min; Drinkwater, Barbara L.; Dishman, RodK.; Mackey, Maureen; Keinholz, Michelle L. Physical Activity, Nutrition, and Chronic Disease. *Medicine and Science in Sports and Exercise: Volume 28(3) March 1996 pp 335-349,* Copyright 2006 American College of Sports Medicine

18. Anthony J. Blazevich, and Anthony Giorgi. Effect of Testosterone Administration and Weight Training on Muscle Architecture. *Medicine and Science in Sports and Exercise: Volume 33(10) 2001 pp 1688-1693,* Copyright 2006 American College of Sports Medicine

19. Blundell, John E,; King, Neil A. Physical Activity and Regulation of Food Intake: Current Evidence. *Medicine and Science in Sports and Exercise: Volume 31(11) Supplement 1 November 1999 pp. S573,* Copyright 2006 American College of Sports Medicine

20. Kara J. Bosher, Jeffrey A. Potteiger, Chris Gennings, Paul E. Luebbers, Keith A. Shannon, and Robynn M. Shannon. Effects of Different Macronutrient Consumption Following A Resistance-Training Session on Fat and Carbohydrate Metabolism. *J. Strength Cond. Res.,* 2004, 18(2), 212-219, Copyright 2004 National Strength and Conditioning Association

21. Megan Brenner, Janet Walberg Rankin, and Don Sebolt. The Effect of Creatine Supplementation During Resistance Training in Women. *J. Strength Cond. Res.,* 2000, 14(2), 207-213, Copyright 2000 National Strength and Conditioning Association

22. Brown, G. A; Reifenrath, T. A.; Uhl, N. L.; King, D. S. Oral Anabolic-Androgenic Supplements During Resistance Training: Effects on Glucose Tolerance , Insulin Action, and Blood Lipids. *Medicine and Science in Sports and Exercise: Volume 31(5) Supplement May 1999 p S266,* Copyright 2006 American College of Sports Medicine

23. Rachel C. Brown, Charlotte M. Cox, and Ailsa Goulding. High - Carbohydrate Versus High Fat Diets: Effect on Body Composition in Trained Cyclists. *Medicine and Science in Sports and Exercise: Volume 32(3) March 2000 pp 690-694,* Copyright 2006 American College of Sports Medicine

24. Rebecca J. Bryant, Jeff Ryder, Paul Martino, Junghoun Kim, and Bruce W. Craig. Effects of Vitamin E and C Supplementation Either Alone or in Combination on Exercise-Induced Lipid Peroxidation in Trained Cyclists. *J. Strength Cond. Res.,* 2003, 17(4), 792-800, Copyright 2003 National Strength and Conditioning Association

25. Buckley, J. D.; Brinkworth, G. D.; Slavotinek, J. P. Effect of Bovine Colostrum Supplementation on The Composition of Resistance Trained and Non-Resistance Rained Limbs. *Medicine and Science in Sports and Exercise: Volume 33(5) Supplement 1 May 2001, p S340,* Copyright 2006 American College of Sports Medicine

26. Louise M. Burke, John A. Hawley, Damien J. Angus, Gregory R. Cox, Sally A. Clark, NicolaK. Cummings, Ben Desbrow, and Mark Hargreaves. Adaptation to Short-Term High-Fat Diet Persist During Exercise Despite High Carbohydrate Availability. *Medicine and Science in Sports and Exercise: Volume 34(1) 2002 pp. 83-91,* Copyright 2006 American College of Sports Medicine

27. Darren G. Burke, Truis Smith-Palmer, Laurence E. Holt, Brian Head, and Phillip D. Chilibeck. The Effect of 7 Days fo Creatine Supplementation on 24-Hour Urinary Creatine Excretion. *J. Strength Cond. Res.,* 2001, 15(1), 59-62, Copyright 2001 National Strength and Conditioning Association

28. Louise M. Burke and John A. Hawley. Effects of Short-Term Fat Adaptation on Metabolism and Performance of Prolonged Exercise. *Medicine and Science in Sports and Exercise: Volume 34(9) 2002 pp. 1492-1498,* Copyright 2006 American College of Sports Medicine

29. Silvia Canete, Alejandro F. San Juan, Margarita Perez, Felix Gomez-Gallego, Luis M. Lopez-Mojares, Conrad P. Earnest, Steven J. Fleck, and Alejandro Lucia. Does Creatine Supplementation Improve Functional Capacity in Elderly Women. *J. Strength Cond. Res.* 20(1), 22-28, 2006 Copyright 2006 National Strength and Conditioning Association

30. Michael A. Clark, Rodney J. Corn. NASM OPT Optimum Performance Training for the Fitness Professional, 2nd Edition. Copyright 2001, National Academy of Sports Medicine.

31. Jared W. Coburn, Dona J. Housh, Terry J Housh, Moh H. Malek, Travis W. Beck, Joel T. Cramer, Glen O. Johnson and Patrick E. Donlin. Effects of Leucine and Whey Protein Supplementation During Eight Weeks of Unilateral Resistance Training. *J. Strength Cond. Res.*, 2006, 20(2), 284-291, Copyright 2006 National Strength and Conditioning Association

32. Eileen G. Collins, W. Edwin Langbein, Cynthia Orebaugh, Christine Bammert, Karla Hanson, Domenic Reda, Lonnie C. Edwards, and Fred N. Littooy. PoleStriding Exercise and Vitamin E for Management of Peripheral Vascular Disease. *Medicine and Science in Sports and Exercise: Volume 35(3) 2003 pp. 384-392,* Copyright 2006 American College of Sports Medicine

33. G. Trevor Cottrell, J. Richard Coast, and Robert A. Herb. Effect of Recovery Interval on Multiple-Bout Sprint Cycling Performance After Acute Creatine Supplementation. *J. Strength Cond. Res.*, 2002, 16(1), 109-116, Copyright 2002 National Strength and Conditioning Association

34. Crespo, Carlos J.; Ainsworth, Barbara E.; Keteyian, Steven J.; Heath, Gregory W.; Smit, Ellen. Prevalence of Physical Inactivity and Its Relation to Social Class in U.S. Adults: Results From the Third National Health and Nutrition Examination Survey, 1988-1994. *Medicine and Science in Sports and Exercise: Volume*

31(12) December1999 pp 1821, Copyright 2006 American College of Sports Medicine

35. Sheree N. Colson, Frank B. Wyatt, Deborah L. Johnston, Lance D. Autrey, Youlanda L. Fitzgerald, and Conrad P. Earnest. Cordyceps Sinensis- and Rhodiola Rosea-Based Supplementation in Male Cyclists and Its Effect on Muscle Tissue Oxygen Saturation. *J. Strength Cond. Res.,* 2005, 19(2), 358-363, Copyright 2005 National Strength and Conditioning Association

36. Brian Dawson, Todd Vladich, and Brian A. Blanksby. Effects of 4 Weeks of Creatine Supplementation in Junior Swimmers on Freestyle Sprint and Swim Bench Performance. *J. Strength Cond. Res.,* 2002, 16(4), 485-490, Copyright 2002 National Strength and Conditioning Association

37. Christophe Delecluse, Rudi Diels, and Marina Goris. Effect of Creatine Supplementation on Intermittent Sprint Running Performance in Highly Trained Athletes. *J. Strength Cond. Res.,* 2003, 17(3), 446-454, Copyright 2003 National Strength and Conditioning Association

38. Keith C. Deruisseau, Lara M. Roberts, Michael R. Kushnik, Allison M. Evans, Krista Austin, and Emily M. Haynes. Iron Status of Young Males and Females Performing Weight-Training Exercise. *Medicine and Science in Sports and Exercise: Volume 36(2) 2004 pp 241-248,* Copyright 2006 American College of Sports Medicine

39. DeSisso, Travis D.; Gerst Jonathan W.; Carnathan, Patrick D.; Kukta, Leslie C.; Skelton, Lauren E.; Bland, Justin R.; Turley, Kenneth R. Effect of Caffeine on Metabolic and Cardiovascular Responses to Submaximal Exercises: Boys Versus Men: 2429 2:00 PM - 2:15 PM *Medicine and Science in Sports and Exercise: Volume 37(5) Supplement May 2005 p. S465,* Copyright 2006 American College of Sports Medicine

40. Di Bello, Vitantonio; Giorgi, Davide; Bianchi, Massimiliano; Bertini, Alessio; Caputo, MariaTeresa; Valenti, Giosue; Furioso, Orlando; Alessandri, Lorenzo; Paterni, Marco Giusti, Costantino. Effects of Anabolic-Androgenic Steroids on Weight-Lifters' Myocardium: An Ultrasonic Videodensitometric Study. *Medicine and Science in Sports and Exercise: Volume 31(4) April 1999 pp 514-521*, Copyright 2006 American College of Sports Medicine

41. Francesco Saverio Dioguardi. Influence of the Ingestion of Branched Chain Amino Acids on Plasma Concentrations of Ammonia and Free Fatty Acids. *J. Strength Cond. Res.*, 1997, 11(4), 242-245, Copyright 1997 National Strength and Conditioning Association

42. Conrad P. Earnest, Stacey L. Lancaster, Christopher J. Rasmussen, Chad M. Kerksick, Alejandro Lucia, Michael C. Greenwood, Anthony L. Almada, Patty A. Cowan, and Richard B. Krieder. Low Vs. High Glycemic Index Carbohydrate Gel Ingestion During Simulated 64-KM Cycling Time Trial Performance. *J. Strength Cond. Res.* 18(3), 466-472, Copyright 2004 National Strength and Conditioning Association

43. Ebbling, Cara B.; Rodriguez, Nancy R. Effects of Exercise Combined With Diet Therapy on Protein Utilization in Obese Children. *Medicine and Science in Sports and Exercise: Volume 31(3) March 1999 pp. 378-385*, Copyright 2006 American College of Sports Medicine

44. Kyle t. Ebersole, Jeffrey R. Stout, Joan M. Eckerson, Terry J. Housh, Tammy K. Evetovich, and Douglas B. Smith. The Effect of Pyruvate Supplementation on Critical Power. *J. Strength Cond. Res.* 14(2), 132-134, 2000, Copyright 2000 National Strength and Conditioning Association

45. Joan M. Eckrson, Jeffrey R. Stout, Geri A. Moore, Nancy J. Stone, Kate A. Iwan, Amy N. Gebauer, and Rachelle Ginsberg. Effect of

Creatine Phosphate Supplementation on Anaerobic Working Capacity and Body Weight After Two and Six Days of Loading in Men and Women. *J. Strength Cond. Res.* 19(4), 756-763, 2005, Copyright 2005 National Strength and Conditioning Association

46. Michael R. Edwards, Edward C. Rhodes, Donald C. McKenzie, and Angelo N. Belcastro. The Effect of Creatine Supplementation on Anaerobic Performance in Moderately Active Men. *J. Strength Cond. Res.*, 2000, 14(1), 75-79, Copyright 2000 National Strength and Conditioning Association

47. Bert Op 'T Eijende and Peter Hespel. Short -Term Creatine Supplementation Does Not Alter The Hormonal Response to Resistance Training. *Medicine and Science in Sports and Exercise: Volume 33(3) 2001 pp 449-453,* Copyright 2006 American College of Sports Medicine

48. Engelhardt, Martin; Neuman, Georg; Berbalk, Annaliese; Reuter, Iris. Creatine Supplementation in Endurance Sports. *Medicine and Science in Sports and Exercise: Volume 30(7) July 1998 pp. 1123-1129,* Copyright 2006 American College of Sports Medicine

49. Herman-J. Engels, Ilektra Kolokouri, Thomas J. Cieslak II, and John C. Wirth. Effects of Ginseng Supplementation on Supramaximal Exercise Performance and Short Term-Recovery. *J. Strength Cond. Res.* 2001, 15(3), 290-295, Copyright 2005 National Strength and Conditioning Association

50. Kelly Anne Erdman, Tak S. Fung, and Raylene A. Reimer. Influence of Performance Level on Dietary Supplementation in Elite Canadian Athletes. *Medicine and Science in Sports and Exercise: Volume 38(2) 2006 pp. 349-356,* Copyright 2006 American College of Sports Medicine

51. Darin J. Falk, Kate A. Heelan, John P. Thyfault, and Alex J. Koch. Effects of Effervescent Creatine, Ribose, and Glutamine

Supplementation on Muscular Strength, Muscular Endurance, and Body Composition. *J. Strength Cond. Res.* 17(4), 810-816, 2003 Copyright 2003 National Strength and Conditioning Association

52. Heather Hedrick Fink, Lisa A. Burgoon, Alan E. Mikesky. Practical Application in Sports Nutrition. Copyright 2006 by Jones and Bartlett Publishers, Inc.

53. Eric W. Finstad, Ian J. Newhouse, Henry C. Lukaski, Jim E. McAuliffe, and Cameron R. Stewart. The Effects of Magnesium Supplementation on Exercise Performance. *Medicine and Science in Sports and Exercise: Volume 33(3) 2001 pp. 493-498,* Copyright 2006 American College of Sports Medicine

54. Flynn, M. G.; Braun, W. A.; Armstrong, J.; Lambert, C. P.; Jacks, D.; Yates, J.; Mylona, E. Effect of Oral Chondroitin Sulfate Supplements on Muscle Soreness, Creatine Kinase, and Markers of Inflammation. *Medicine and Science in Sports and Exercise: Volume 30(5) Supplement May 1998 p. 103,* Copyright 2006 American College of Sports Medicine

55. Fogelholm, Mikael; Hilloskorpi, Hannele. Weight and Diet Concerns in Finnish Female and Male Athletes. *Medicine and Science in Sports and Exercise: Volume 31(2) February 1999 pp. 229-235,* Copyright 2006 American College of Sports Medicine

56. Gaesser, Glenn A. Thinness and Weight Loss: Beneficial or Detrimental to Longevity? *Medicine and Science in Sports and Exercise: Volume 31(8) August 1999 pp. 1118-1128,* Copyright 2006 American College of Sports Medicine

57. Kara J. Gallagher, John M. Jakicic, Melissa A. Napolitano, and Bess H. Marcus. Psychological Factors Related to Physical Activity and Weight Loss in Overweight Women. *Medicine and Science*

in Sports and Exercise: Volume 38(5) 2006 pp. 971-980, Copyright 2006 American College of Sports Medicine

58. Philip M. Gallagher, John A. Carrithers, Michael P. Godard, Kimberley E. Schulze, and Scott W. Trappe. B-Hydroxy-B-Methylbutyrate Ingestion, Part I: Effects on Strength and Fat Free Mass. *Medicine and Science in Sports and Exercise: Volume 32(12) 2000 pp. 2109-2115,* Copyright 2006 American College of Sports Medicine

59. Mark Glaister, Richard A. Lockey, Corinne S. Abraham, Allan Staerck, Jon E. Goodwin, and Gillian McInnes. Creatine Supplementation and Multiple Sprint Running Performance. *J. Strength Cond. Res.* 20(2), 273-277, Copyright 2006 National Strength and Conditioning Association

60. J. Matt Green, John R. McLester, Jr., Joe E. Smith, and Edward R. Mansfield. The Effects of Creatine Supplementation on Repeated Upper- and Lower-Body Wingate Performance. *J. Strength Cond. Res.,* 2001, 15(1), 36-41, Copyright 2001 National Strength and Conditioning Association

61. Gutgessell, Margaret E.; Timmerman, Mark; Keller, Adrienne. Reported Alcohol Use and Behavior in Long Distance Runners. *Medicine and Science in Sports and Exercise: Volume 28(8) August 1996 pp. 1063-1070,* Copyright 2006 American College of Sports Medicine

62. G. Gregory Haff, Michael H. Stone, Beverly J. Warren, Robert Keith, Robert L. Johnson, David C. Nieman, Franklin Williams Jr., and K. Brett Kirsky. The Effect of Carbohydrate Supplementation Multiple Sessions and Bouts of Resistance Training. *J. Strength Cond. Res.* 13(2), 111-117, Copyright 1995 National Strength and Conditioning Association

63. G. Gregory Haff, K. Brett Kirsky. Michael H. Stone, Beverly J. Warren, Robert L. Johnson, Meg Stone, Harold O'Bryant, and Chris Poulx The Effect of 6-Weeks of Creatine Monohydrate Supplementation on Dynamic Rate of Force Development. *J. Strength Cond. Res.*, 2000, 14(4), 426-433, Copyright 2000 National Strength and Conditioning Association

64. G. Gregory Haff, Mark J. Lehmkuhl, Lora B. McCoy, and Michael H. Stone. Carbohydrate Supplementation and Resistance Training. *J. Strength Cond. Res.* 17(1), 187-196, Copyright 2003 National Strength and Conditioning Association

65. John A. Hawley.   Effect of Increased Fat Availability on Metabolism and Exercise Capacity. *Medicine and Science in Sports and Exercise: Volume 34(9) 2002 pp. 1485-1491,* Copyright 2006 American College of Sports Medicine

66. Hefferan T.E.; Kennedy A.M.; Evans G.L.; Turner R.T. Disuse Exaggerates the Detrimental Effects of Alcohol on Cortical Bone. Alcohol Clin Exp Res. 2003 Jan;27(1): 111-7
http://www.ncbl.nlm.nih.gov/entrez/query.fcgi?cmd=Retrieve&db=PubMed&list_uids=12...

67. Helge, Jorn W.; Wulff, Bilette; Kiens, Bente. Impact of a Fat-Rich Diet on Endurance in Man: Role of The Dietary Period. *Medicine and Science in Sports and Exercise: Volume 30(3) March 1998 pp. 456-461,* Copyright 2006 American College of Sports Medicine

68. Jorn Wulff Helge. Long-Term fat diet adaptation effects on performance, training capacity, and fat utilization. *Medicine and Science in Sports and Exercise: Volume 34(9) p. 1499-1504,* Copyright 2002 American College of Sports Medicine

69. Jay R. Hoffman, Jeffrey R. Stout, Michael J. Falvo, Jie Kang, and Nicholas A. Ratamess.   Effect of Low-Dose, Short Duration Creatine Supplementation on Anaerobic Exercise Performance.

J. Strength Cond. Res., 2005 19(2), 260-264, Copyright 2005 National Strength and Conditioning Association

70. Harri Hemila, Jarmo Viramo, Demetrius Albanes, and Jaakko Kaprio. Physical Activity and the Common Cold in Men Administered Vitamin E and B-Carotene. *Medicine and Science in Sports and Exercise: Volume 35(11) 2003 pp. 1815-1820,* Copyright 2006 American College of Sports Medicine

71. Edward T. Howley, B. Don Franks. Health Fitness Instructors Handbook - 3rd Edition. Human Kinetics, Copyright 1997, 1992, 1986 by Edward T. Howley and B. Don Franks

72. Juha J. Hulmi, Jeff S. Volek, Harri Selanne, and Antti A. Mero. Protein Ingestion Prior to Strength Exercise Affects Blood Hormones and Metabolism. *Medicine and Science in Sports and Exercise: Volume 37(11) November 2005 pp 1990-1997,* Copyright 2006 American College of Sports Medicine

73. Gary R. Hunter and Nuala M. Byrne. Physical Activity and Muscle Function but Not Resting Energy Expenditure Impact on Weight Gain. *J. Strength Cond. Res.* 19(1), 225-230, Copyright 2005 National Strength and Conditioning Association

74. Bert H. Jacobson and Hugh A. Gemmell. Nutrition Information Sources of College Varsity Athletes. *Journal of Applied Sport Science and Research.*, 1991, 5(4), 204-207, Copyright 1991 National Strength and Conditioning Association

75. Bert H. Jacobson and Steven G. Aldana. Current Nutrition Practice and Knowledge of Varsity Athletes. *Journal of Applied Sport Science and Research*, 1992, 6(4), 232-238, Copyright 1992 National Strength and Conditioning Association

76. Bert H. Jacobson, Chris Sobonya, and Jack Ransone. Nutrition Practices and Knowledge of College Varsity Athletes: A

Follow-Up. *J. Strength Cond. Res.*,2001, 15(1), 63-68, Copyright 2001 National Strength and Conditioning Association

77. Jakicic, John M.; Polley, Betsy A.; Wing, Rena R. Accuracy of Self Reported Exercise and the Relationship With Weight Loss in Overweight Women. *Medicine and Science in Sports and Exercise: Volume 30(4) April 1998 pp. 634-638*, Copyright 2006 American College of Sports Medicine

78. John M. Jakicic, Rena W. Wing, and Carena Winters-Hart. Relationship of Physical Activity to Eating Behaviors and Weight Loss in Women. *Medicine and Science in Sports and Exercise: Volume 34(10) October 2002 pp 1653-1659*, Copyright 2006 American College of Sports Medicine

79. Mark Jarvis, Lars McNaughton, Alan Seddon, and Dylan Thompson. The Acute 1-Week Effects of the Zone Diet on Body Composition, Blood Lipid Levels, and Performance in Recreational Endurance Athletes. *J. Strength Cond. Res.* 16(1) 2002, 50-57, Copyright 2002 National Strength and Conditioning Association

80. Roy L. P. G. Jentjens, Juul Achten, and Asker Jeukendrup. High Oxidation Rates from Combined Carbohydrate Ingested During Exercise. *Medicine and Science in Sports and Exercise: Volume 36(9) 2004 pp. 1551-1558*, Copyright 2006 American College of Sports Medicine

81. Vincent G. Kelly and David G. Jenkins. Effect of Oral Creatine Supplementation on Near-Maximal Strength and Repeated Sets of High-Intensity Bench Press Exercise. *J. Strength Cond. Res.*, 1998, 12(2), 109-115, Copyright 1998 National Strength and Conditioning Association

82. King, D. S.; Sharp, R. L.; Brown, G. A.; Reifenrath, T. A.; Uhl, N. L. Oral Anabolic-Androgenic Supplements During Resistance Training:

Effects on Serum Testosterone and Estrogen Concentrations. *Medicine and Science in Sports and Exercise: Volume 31(5) Supplement May 1999 p S266,* Copyright 2006 American College of Sports Medicine

83. Brett Kirsky, Michael H. Stone, Beverly J. Warren, Robert L. Johnson, Meg Stone, G. Gregory Hafe, Franklin E. Williams, and Christopher Poulx. The Effects of 6 Weeks of Creatine Monohydrate Supplementation on Performance Measures and Body Composition in Collegiate Track and Field Athletes. *J. Strength Cond. Res.,* 1999, 13(2), 148-156, Copyright 1999 National Strength and Conditioning Association

84. William J. Kraemer, Jeff S. Volek, Duncan N. French, Martyn R. Rubin, Matthew J. Sharman, Ana L. Gomez, Nicholas A. Ratamess, Robert U. Newton, Bozena Jemiolo, Bruce W. Craig, and Keijo Hakkinen. The Effects of L-Carnitine L-Tartrate Supplementation on Hormonal Responses to Resistance Exercise and Recovery. *J. Strength Cond. Res.,* 2003, 17(3), 455-462, Copyright 2003 National Strength and Conditioning Association

85. Kraemer, William J.; Volek, Jeff S.; Clark, Kristin L.; Gordon, Scott E.; Puhl, Susan M.; Koziris, L. Perry; McBride, Jeffrey M.; Triplett-McBride, N. Travis; Putukian, Margot; Newton, Robert U.; Hakkinen, Keijo; Bush, Jill A.; Sebastianelli, Wayne J.. Influence of Exercise Training on Physiological and Performance Changes With Weight Loss in Men. *Medicine and Science in Sports and Exercise: Volume 31(9) September 1999 pp. 1320-1329,* Copyright 2006 American College of Sports Medicine

86. Kreider, Richard B.; Ferreira, Maria; Wilson, Michael; Grindstaff, Pamela; Plisk, Steven; Reinardy, Jeff; Cantler, Edward; Almada, A. L. Effects of Creatine Supplementation on Body Composition, Strength, and Sprint Performance. *Medicine and Science in Sports and Exercise: Volume 30(1) January 1998 pp. 73-82,* Copyright 2006 American College of Sports Medicine

87. Richard B. Kreider, Maria P. Ferreira, Michael Greenwood, Michael Wilson, and Anthony L. Almada. Effects of Conjugated Linoleic Acid Supplementation During Resistance Training on Body Composition, Bone Density, Strength, and Selected Hematological Markers. *J. Strength Cond. Res.*, 2002, 16(3), 325-334, Copyright 2002 National Strength and Conditioning Association

88. Matthew R. Kutz and Michael J. Gunter. Creatine Monohydrate Supplementation on Body Weight and Percent Body Fat. *J. Strength Cond. Res.*, 2003, 17(4), 817-821, Copyright 2003 National Strength and Conditioning Association

89. Laitinen J.; Pietilainen K.; Wadsworth M.; Sovia U.; Jarvelin MR. Predictors of Abdominal Obesity Among 31-y-old Men and Women Born in Northern Finland in 1966. *Eur J Clin Nutr. 2004 Jan: 58(1): 180-90*
http://www.ncbl.nlm.nih.gov/entrez/query.fcgi?cmd=Retreive&db=PubMed&list_uids=14...

90. Kotcha Larew, Gary R. Hunter, D. Ennete Larson-Meyer, Bradley R. Newcomer, John P. McCarthy, and Roland L. Weinser. Muscle Metabolic Function, Exercise Performance, and Weight Gain. *Medicine and Science in Sports and Exercise: Volume 35(2) pp. 230-236, 2003*, Copyright 2006 American College of Sports Medicine

91. D. Ennette Larson-Meyer, Gary R. Hunter, Christina A. Throwbridge, Joanne C. Turk, James M. Ernest, Stacey L. Torman, and Paul A. Harbin. The Effect of Creatine Supplementation on Muscle Strength and Body Composition During Off-Season Training in Female Soccer Players.

92. Leddy, John; Horvath, Peter; Rowland, Jill; Pendergast, David. Effect of a High or a Low Fat Diet on Cardiovascular Risk Factors in Male and Female Runners. *Medicine and Science in Sports and*

Exercise: Volume 29(1) January 1997 pp17-25, Copyright 2006 American College of Sports Medicine

93. Ashleigh Ledford and John David Branch. Creatine Supplementation Does Not Increase Peak Power Production and Work Capacity During Repetitive Wingate Testing in Women. *J. Strength Cond. Res.*, 1999, 13(4), 394-399, Copyright 1999 National Strength and Conditioning Association

94. Mark Lehmkuhl, Molly Malone, Blake Justice, Greg Trone, Ed Pistilli, Debra Vinci, Erin E. Haff, J. Lon Kilgore, and G. Gregory Haff. The Effects of 8 Weeks of Creatine Monohydrate and Glutamine. *J. Strength Cond. Res.*, 2000, 14(4), 434-442, Copyright 2000 National Strength and Conditioning Association

95. Supplementation on Body Composition and Performance Measures. *J. Strength Cond. Res.*, 2003, 17(3), 425-438, Copyright 2003 National Strength and Conditioning Association

96. Michael Leveritt and Peter J. Abernethy. Effects of Carbohydrate Restrictions on Strength Performance. *J. Strength Cond. Res. 13(1) pp.52-57* Copyright 2006 National Strength and Conditioning Association

97. Liang, Michael T.; Moreno, Alejandro M.; Young Lisa K.; Chaung, William. Effects of Panaz Notoginseng on Aerobic Endurance and Cardiovascular Parameters in Adult Humans: 220 Board #127 9:30AM - 11:00AM. *Medicine and Science in Sports and Exercise: Volume 37(5) Supplement May 2005 p. S41*, Copyright 2006 American College of Sports Medicine

98. Lindeman, Alice K. Quest for Ideal Weight: Costs and Consequences. *Medicine and Science in Sports and Exercise: Volume 31(8) 1999 pp. 1135-1140*, Copyright 2006 American College of Sports Medicine

99. Lovell, Richard J.; Pout, Martin J.; Ryder, James J. Beverage Temperature: Effects upon Cardiovascular and Thermoregulatory Responses to Endurance Activity. *Medicine and Science in Sports and Exercise: Volume 36(5) Supplement May 2004 p. S315,* Copyright 2006 American College of Sports Medicine

100. MacTaggart, J. N., Hansen, M. R.; Kolhorst, F. W. Effect of the Access Fat Conversion Activity Bar on Fat Utilization and Time to Exhaustion 292. *Medicine and Science in Sports and Exercise: Volume 29(5) Supplement 1 May 1997 p. S342,* Copyright 2006 American College of Sports Medicine

101. Meir Magal, Michael J. Webster, Lucille E. Sistrunk, Malcolm T. Whitehead, Ronald K. Evans, Joseph C. Boyd. Comparison of Glycerol and Water Hydration Regimens on Tennis-Related Performance. *Medicine and Science in Sports and Exercise: Volume 35(1) p. 150-156, 2003* Copyright 2006 American College of Sports Medicine

102. Malloy-McFall, J: Dochstander, L; Otterstetter, R; Lowery, L; Ziegenfuss, T; Caine, N; Glickman, E.L. Effect of an Herbal Supplement on Thermoregulatory, Cardiovascular, and Metabolic Responses During Submaximal Exercise. *Medicine and Science in Sports and Exercise: Volume 34(5) Supplement 1 May 2002 p. S225,* Copyright 2006 American College of Sports Medicine

103. Melissa J. Mayo, Justin R. Grantham, and Govindasamy Balasekaren. Exercise-Induced Weight Loss Preferentially Reduces Abdominal Fat. *Medicine and Science in Sports and Exercise: Volume 35(2) February 2003 pp 207-213,* Copyright 2006 American College of Sports Medicine

104. Sasa Mihic, Jay R. MacDonald, Scott McKenzie, and Mark A. Tarnopolsky. Acute Creatine Loading Increases Fat-Free Mass, but Does Not Affect Blood Pressure, Plasma Creatinine, or CK

Activity in Men and Women. *Medicine and Science in Sports and Exercise: Volume 32(2) February 2000 pp. 291-296,* Copyright 2006 American College of Sports Medicine

105. Miller, Wayne C. How Effective are Traditional Dietary and Exercise Interventions for Weight Loss? *Medicine and Science in Sports and Exercise: Volume 31(8) August 1999 pp. 129-1134,* Copyright 2006 American College of Sports Medicine

106. Miro, A. A.; Nykanen, T.; Rasi, S.; Leppaluoto, J. IGF-1, IGFBP-3, Growth Hormone and Testosterone in Male and Female Athletes During Bovine Colostrum Supplementation. *Medicine and Science in Sports and Exercise: Volume 34(5) Supplement 1 May 2002 p. S299,* Copyright 2006 American College of Sports Medicine

107. Antti A. Miro, Kari L. Keskinen, Marko T. Malvela, and Janne M. Sallinen. Combined Creatine and Sodium Bicarbonate Supplementation Enhances Interval Swimming. *J. Strength Cond. Res.,* 2004, 18(2), 306-310, Copyright 2004 National Strength and Conditioning Association Joel B. Mitchell, Jonathan P. Dugas, Brian K. McFarlin and Matthew J. Nelson. Effect of Exercise, Heat Stress, and Hydration on Immune Cell Number and Function. *Medicine and Science in Sports and Exercise: Volume 34(12) 2002 p. 1941-1950,*Copyright 2006 American College of Sports Medicine

108. Mittleman, Karen D.; Ricci, Matthew R.; Bailey, Stephen P. Branched-Chain Amino Acids Prolong Exercise During Heat Stress in Men and Women. *Medicine and Science in Sports and Exercise: Volume 30(1) January 1998 pp 83-91,* Copyright 2006 American College of Sports Medicine

109. Mujika, Inigo; Chatard, Jean-Claude; Lacoste, Lucien; Barale, Frederic; Geyssant, Andre. Creatine Supplementation Does Not Improve Sprint Performance in Competitive Swimmers. *Medicine and Science in Sports and Exercise: Volume 28(11)*

November 1996 pp 1435-1441, Copyright 2006 American College of Sports Medicine

110. Inigo Mujik, Sabino Padilla, Javier Ibanez, Mikel Izquerdo, and Esteban Garostiaga. Creatine Supplementation and Sprint Performance in Soccer Platers. *Medicine and Science in Sports and Exercise: Volume 32(2) 2000 pp. 518-525,* Copyright 2006 American College of Sports Medicine

111. Arnold G. Nelson, David A. Arnall, Joke Kokkenen, Randy Day, and Jared Evans. Muscle Glycogen Supercompensation is Enhanced by Prior Creatine Supplementation. *Medicine and Science in Sports and Exercise: Volume 33(7) July 2001 pp. 1096-1100,* Copyright 2006 American College of Sports Medicine

112. Toben F. Nelson and Henry Wechsler. Alcohol and College Athletes. *J. Strength Cond. Res.* 33(1), 43-47, Copyright 2001 National Strength and Conditioning Association

113. Laura E. Newton, Gary Hunter, Mark Bammon, and Robin Roney. Changes in Psychological State and Self-Reported Diet During Various Phases of Training ion Competitive Bodybuilders. *J. Strength Cond. Res.* 7(3), 153-158, Copyright 1993 National Strength and Conditioning Association

114. Davdid C. Nieman, Dru A. Henson, Steven R. McAnulty, Lisa S. McAnulty, Jason D. Morrow, Alaa Ahmed, and Chris B. Heward. Vitamin E and Immunity After the Kona Triathlon World Championship. *Medicine and Science in Sports and Exercise: Volume 36(8) 2004 pp. 1328-1335,* Copyright 2006 American College of Sports Medicine

115. Nindl, Bradley C.; Freidl, Karl E.; Marchitelli, Louis J.; Shippee, Ronald L.; Thomas, Cecilia D.: Patton, John F.. Regional Fat Placement in Physically Fit Males and Changes With Weight Loss. *Medicine and Science in Sports and Exercise: Volume 28(7) July*

1996 pp. 786-793, Copyright 2006 American College of Sports Medicine

116. Odland, L. Maureen; MacDougall, J. Duncan; Tarnopolsky, Mary A.; Elorriaga, A.; Borgmann, Anne. Effect of Oral Creatine Supplementation on Muscle [PCr] and Short-Term Maximum Power Output. *Medicine and Science in Sports and Exercise: Volume 29(2) February 1997 pp. 216-219,* Copyright 2006 American College of Sports Medicine

117. Okano, Goroh; Sato, Yuji; Murata, Yoshihisa. Effect of Elevated Blood FFA Levels on Endurance Performance After a Single Fat Meal Ingestion. *Medicine and Science in Sports and Exercise: Volume 30(5) May 1998 pp. 763-768,* Copyright 2006 American College of Sports Medicine

118. Stephen K. Oliver, and Mark S. Tremblay. Effects of a Sports Nutrition Bar on Endurance Running Performance. *J. Strength Cond. Res.* 16(1), 152-156, Copyright 2002 National Strength and Conditioning Association

119. Parkin, Jo Ann M.; Carey, Michael F.; Martin Iva K.; Stojanovska, Lillian; Febbraio, Mark A.. Muscle Glycogen Storage Following Prolonged Exercise: Effect of Timing of Ingestion of High Glycemic Index Foods. *Medicine and Science in Sports and Exercise: Volume 29(2) February 1997 pp. 220-224,* Copyright 2006 American College of Sports Medicine

120. Portmans, Jacques R.; Francaux, Mark. Long-Term Oral Creatine Supplementation Does Not Impair Renal Function in Healthy Athletes. *Medicine and Science in Sports and Exercise: Volume 31(8) August 1999 pp. 1108-1110,* Copyright 2006 American College of Sports Medicine

121. Eric S. Rawson, Bridget Gunn, and Priscilla M. Clarkson. The Effects of Creatine Supplementation on Exercise-Induced Muscle

Damage. *J. Strength Cond. Res.*, 2001, 15(2), 178-184, Copyright 2001 National Strength and Conditioning Association

122. Eric S. Rawson, Adam M. Perky, Thomas B. Price, and Priscilla M. Clarkson. Effects of Repeated Creatine Supplementation on Muscle, Plasma, and Urine Creatine Levels. *J. Strength Cond. Res.*, 2004, 18(1), 162-167, Copyright 2004 National Strength and Conditioning Association

123. Eric S. Rawson, and Jeff S. Vole. Effects of Creatine Supplementation and Resistance Training on Muscle Strength and Weight Lifting Performance. *J. Strength Cond. Res.*, 2003, 17(4), 822-831, Copyright 2003 National Strength and Conditioning Association

124. Reed, A.H.; McCarty, H.L.; Evans, G.L.; Turner, R.T.; Westerland, K.C. The Effects of Chronic Alcohol Consumption and Exercise on the Skeleton of Adult Male Rats. Alcohol Clin Exp Res. 2002 Aug;26(8): 1269-74
http://www.ncbl.nlm.nih.gov/entrez/query.fcgi?cmd=Retrieve&db=PubMed&list_uids=12...

125. John A. Rockwell, Janet Walberg Rankin, and Ben Toderico. Creatine Supplementation Affects Muscle Creatine During Energy Restriction. *Medicine and Science in Sports and Exercise: Volume 33(1) 2001 pp 61-68,* Copyright 2006 American College of Sports Medicine

126. Ross, Robert; Janssen, Ian. Is Abdominal Fat Preferentially Reduced in Response to Exercise-Induced Weight Loss? *Medicine and Science in Sports and Exercise: Volume 31(11) Supplement 1 November 1999 p. S568,* Copyright 2006 American College of Sports Medicine

127. Rowland, Thomas W.; Pober, David; Garrison, Anne. Determinants of Cardiovascular Drift in Euhydrated Prepubertal Boys: 1146

Board #1. *Medicine and Science in Sports and Exercise: Volume 37(5) Supplement May 2005 p. S216,* Copyright 2006 American College of Sports Medicine

128. Scanga, Connie B.; Verde, Tony J.; Paolone, Albert M.; Anderson, Ross E.; Wadden, Thomas A. Effects of Weight Loss and Exercise Training on Natural Killer Cell Activity in Obese Women. *Medicine and Science in Sports and Exercise: Volume 30(12) December 1998 pp. 1666-1671,* Copyright 2006 American College of Sports Medicine

129. Timothy C. Schell, Glen Wright, Paul Martino, Jeff Ryder, and Bruce W. Craig. Postexercise Glucose, Insulin, and C-Peptide Responses to Carbohydrate Supplementation: Running vs. Resistance Exercise. *J. Strength Cond. Res.* 13(4), 372-380, Copyright 1999 National Strength and Conditioning Association

130. Brian K. Schilling, Michael H. Stone, Alan Utter, Jay T. Kearney, Mary Johnson, Robert Coglianese, Lucille Smith, Harold S. O'Bryant, Andrew C. Fry, Mike Starks, Robert Keith, Margaret E. Stone. Creatine Supplementation and Health Variables: A Retrospective Study. *Medicine and Science in Sports and Exercise: Volume 33(2) 2001, pp. 183-188,* Copyright 2001 American College of Sports Medicine

131. Schmid, Andreas; Jakob, Ernst; Berg, Aloys; Rumann, Thomas; Konig, Daniel; Irmer, Manfred; Keul, Joseph. Effect of Physical Exercise and Vitamin C on Absorption of Ferric Sodium Citrate. *Medicine and Science in Sports and Exercise: Volume 28(12) December 1996 pp 1470-1473,* Copyright 2004 American College of Sports Medicine

132. Joshua T. Selsby, Robert A. DiSilvestro, and Steven T. Devor. Mg2+-Creatine Chelate and A Low-Dose Creatine Supplementation Regimen Improve Exercise Performance. *J. Strength Cond. Res.,*

2004, 18(2), 311-315, Copyright 2004 National Strength and Conditioning Association

133. Sisngh, Anita; Papanicolaou, Dimitris, A.; Lawrence, Linda L.; Howell, Elise A.; Chrousos, Goerge P. Deuster, Patricia A.. Neuroendocrine Responses to Running in Women after Zinc and Vitamin Supplementation. *Medicine and Science in Sports and Exercise: Volume 31(4) 1999 pp. 536-542*, Copyright 2006 American College of Sports Medicine

134. Sharman, M. J.; Volek, J. S.; Fleming, J.; Love, D. M.; Avery, N. G.; Gomez, A. L.; Kraemer, W. J. Exercise Performance Responses to a Ketogenic Diet. *Medicine and Science in Sports and Exercise: Volume 34(5) Supplement 1 May 2002 p S234*, Copyright 2006 American College of Sports Medicine

135. Parco M. Siu, Stephen H.S Wong, John G. Morris, Ching W. Lam, Pak K Chung, and Susan Chung. Effect of Frequency of Carbohydrate Feedings on Recovery and Subsequent Endurance Run. *Medicine and Science in Sports and Exercise: Volume 36(2) p. 315-323*, Copyright 2004 American College of Sports Medicine

136. Gary J., Anthony J. Rice, Ken Sharpe, Rebecca Tanner, David Jenkins, Christopher J. Gore, and Allan G. Hann. Impact of Acute Weight Loss and /or Thermal Stress on Rowing Ergometer Performance. *J. Strength Cond. Res.* 37(8), 1387-1394, Copyright 2005 National Strength and Conditioning Association

137. Nicholas A. Ratamess, William J. Kraemer, Jeff S. Volek, Martyn R. Rubin, Ana L. Gomez, Duncan N. French, Matthew J. Sharman, Michael M. McGuigan, Timothy Scheet, Keijo Hakkinen, Robert U. Newton, and Francisco Dioguardi. The Effects of Amino Acid Supplementation on Muscular Performance During Resistance Training Overreaching. *J. Strength Cond. Res.*, 2003, 17(2), 250-258 Copyright 2003 National Strength and Conditioning Association

138. Starling, Raymond D.; Trappe, Todd A.; Short, Kevin R.; Sheffield-Moore, Melinda; Jozsi, Alison C.; Fink, Williams J.; Costill, David L. Effect of Inosine Supplementation on Aerobic and Anaerobic Cycling Performance. *Medicine and Science in Sports and Exercise: Volume 28(9) 1996 pp. 1193-1198,* Copyright 2006 American College of Sports Medicine

139. Michael J. Saunders, Mark D. Kane, and M. Kent Todd. Effects of a Carbohydrate-Protein Beverage on Cycling Endurance and Muscle Damage. *Medicine and Science in Sports and Exercise: Volume 28(11) November 1996 pp 1435-1441,* Copyright 2006 American College of Sports Medicine

140. Patrick R. Steffen, Andrew Sherwood, Elizabeth C. D. Gullette, Anastasia Georgiades, Alan Hinderliter, and James A Blumenthal. Effects of Exercise and Weight Loss on Blood Pressure During Daily Life. *Medicine and Science in Sports and Exercise: Volume 36(7) 2004 pp. 1233-1238,* Copyright 2006 American College of Sports Medicine

141. Nigel K. Stepto, Andrew L. Carey, Heidi M. Staudacher, Nicola K. Cummings, Louise M. Burke, and John A. Hawley. Effect of Short-Term Fat Adaptation on High Intensity Training. *Medicine and Science in Sports and Exercise: Volume 34(3) March 2002 pp. 449-455,* Copyright 2006 American College of Sports Medicine

142. Jeffrey R. Stout, Joan M. Eckerson, Terry J. Housh, and Kyle T. Ebersole. The Effects of Creatine Supplementation on Anaerobic Working Capacity. *J. Strength Cond. Res.,* 1999, 13(2), 135-138, Copyright 1999 National Strength and Conditioning Association

143. Lori Swirzinski, Richard W. Latin, Kris Berg, and Ann Grandjean. A Survey of Sport Nutrition Supplements in High School Football Players. *J. Strength Cond. Res.,* 2000, 14(1), 464-469, Copyright 2000 National Strength and Conditioning Association

144. Daniel G. Syrotuik, Gordon J. Bell, Robert Burnham, Lorraine L. Sim, Robert A. Calvert, and Ian M. MacLean. Absolute and Relative Strength Performance Following Creatine Monohydrate Supplementation Combined With Periodized Resistance Training. *J. Strength Cond. Res.*, 2000, 14(2), 182-190, Copyright 2000 National Strength and Conditioning Association

145. Pedro J. Teixeira, Scott B. Going, Linda B. Houtkooper, Ellen C. Cussler, Lauve L. Metcalfe, Rob M. Blew, Luis B. Sardinha, and Timothy J. Lohman. Exercise Motivation, Eating, and Body Image Variables as Predictors of Weight Control. *Medicine and Science in Sports and Exercise: Volume 38(1) 2006 pp. 179-188,* Copyright 2006 American College of Sports Medicine

146. Tsintzas, Orestis-Konstantinos; Williams, Clyde; Wilson, Wendy; Burrin, Jackie. Influence of Carbohydrate Supplementation Early in Exercise on Endurance Running Capacity. *Medicine and Science in Sports and Exercise: Volume 28(11) November 1996 pp. 1373-1379,* Copyright 2006 American College of Sports Medicine

147. Twisk, J. W. R.; Mechelen, W.; Kemper, H.C.G. Physical Activity and Physical Fitness During Adolescence and Cardiovascular Risk Factors at Adult Age. *Medicine and Science in Sports and Exercise: Volume 34(5) Supplement 1 May 2002 p. S254,* Copyright 2006 American College of Sports Medicine

148. U.S. Department of Agriculture, Popular Weight Loss diets, White Paper/ January 10, 2001
http://www.lib.umich.edu/govdocs/diet.html

149. Alan C. Utter, Jie Kang, David C. Nieman, Victor A. Brown, Charles L. Dumke, Steve R. McAnulty, and Lisa M. McAnulty. Carbohydrate Supplementation and Perceived Exertion During Resistance Exercise. *J. Strength Cond. Res.* 19(4), 939-943, Copyright 2005 National Strength and Conditioning Association

150. Venktraman, Jaya T.; Pendergast, David. Effects of the Level of Dietary Intake and Endurance Exercise on Plasma Cytokines in Runners. *Medicine and Science in Sports and Exercise: Volume 30(8) August 1998 pp 1198-1204,* Copyright 2006 American College of Sports Medicine

151. Vergauven, Lieven; Brouns, Fred; Hespel, Peter. Carbohydrate Supplementation Improves Stroke Performance in Tennis. *Medicine and Science in Sports and Exercise: Volume 30(8) August 1998 pp. 1289-1295,* Copyright 2006 American College of Sports Medicine

152. Jakob L. Vingren, Lymperis P. Koziris, Scott E. Gordon, William J. Kraemer, Russel T. Turner, and Kim C. Westerland. Chronic Alcohol Intake, Resistance Training, and Muscle Androgen Receptor Content. *J. Strength Cond. Res.* 37(11), 1842-1848, Copyright 2005 National Strength and Conditioning Association

153. Virk, Ricky S.; Dunton, Nancy J.; Young, Jenny C.; Leklem, James E.. Effect of Vitamin B-6 Supplementation on Fuels, Catecholamines, and Amino Acids During Exercise in Men. *Medicine and Science in Sports and Exercise: Volume 31(3) March 1999 pp 400-408,* Copyright 2006 American College of Sports Medicine

154. Richard A. Vogel, Micahael J. Webster, Loran D. Erdmann, and Roger D. Clark. Creatine Supplementation: Effect on Supramaximal Exercise Performance at Two Levels of Acute Hypohydration. *J. Strength Cond. Res.,* 2000, 14(2), 214-219, Copyright 2000 National Strength and Conditioning Association

155. Michael Vogt, Adrian Puntschart, Hans Howland, Bruno Mueller, Christoph Mannhart, Liliane Gfeller, Primus Mullis, and Hans Hoppeler. Effects of Dietary Fat on Muscle Substrates, Metabolism, and Performance in Athletes. *Medicine and Science in Sports and Exercise: Volume 35(6) 2003 pp. 952-960,* Copyright 2006 American College of Sports Medicine

156. Jeff S. Volek. Influence of Nutrition on Responses to Resistance Training. *Medicine and Science in Sports and Exercise: Volume 36(4) April 2004 pp 689-696,* Copyright 2006 American College of Sports Medicine

157. Jeff S. Volek, Mark Boetes, Jill A. Bush, Margot Putukian, Wayne J. Sebastianelli, and William J. Kraemer. Response of Testosterone and Cortisol Concentrations to High Intensity Resistance Exercise Following Creatine Supplementation. *J. Strength Cond. Res.* 11(3), 182-187, Copyright 1997 National Strength and Conditioning Association

158. Volek, Jeff, S.; Duncan, Noel D.; Mazzetti, Scott A.; Staron, Robert S.; Putukian, Margot; Gomez, Ana L.; Pearson, David R.; Fink, William J.; Kraemer, William J.. Performance and Muscle Fiber Adaptations to Creatine Supplementation and Heavy Resistance Training. *Medicine and Science in Sports and Exercise: Volume 31(8) August 1999 pp 1147-1156,* Copyright 2006 American College of Sports Medicine

159. Jeff S. Volek and William J. Kraemer. Creatine Supplementation: Its Effect on Human Muscular Performance and Body Composition. *J. Strength Cond. Res.* 10(3), 200-210, Copyright 1996 National Strength and Conditioning Association

160. Susan B. Votruba, Richard L. Atkinson, Matt D. Hirvonen, and Dale A. Schoeller. Prior Exercise Increases Subsequent Utilization of Dietary Fat. *Medicine and Science in Sports and Exercise: Volume 34(11) November 2002 pp 1757-1765,* Copyright 2006 American College of Sports Medicine

161. Wallace, M. Brian; Lim, Jon; Cutler, Andrew; Bucci, Luke. Effects of Dehydroepiandrosterone vs. Androstenedione Supplements in Men. *Medicine and Science in Sports and Exercise: Volume 31(12) December 1999 pp 1788,* Copyright 2006 American College of Sports Medicine

162. John P. Warber, William J. Tharion, John F. Patton, Catherine M. Champagne, Peter Mitotti, and Harris R. Lieberman. The Effect of Creatine Monohydrate Supplementation on Obstacle Course and Multiple Bench Press Performance. *J. Strength Cond. Res.*, 2002, 16(4), 500-508, Copyright 2003 National Strength and Conditioning Association

163. Mark L. Watsford, Aron J. Murphy, Warwick L. Spinks, and Anderew D. Walshe. Creatine Supplementation and Its Effect on Musculotendinous Stiffness and Performance. *J. Strength Cond. Res.*, 2003, 17(1), 26-33, Copyright 2003 National Strength and Conditioning Association

164. Michael J. Webster. Dietary Supplementation: Effect on Acid-Base Status and Power Output During Repeated Bouts of Supramaximal Exercise. *J. Strength Cond. Res.*, 1997, 11(3), 168-173, Copyright 1997 National Strength and Conditioning Association

165. Yitzhak Weinstein, Tamir Kamerman, Elliot Berry, and Bareket Falk. Mechanical Efficiency of Normal-Weight Prepubertal Boys Predisposed to Obesity. *Medicine and Science in Sports and Exercise: Volume 36(4) pp. 567-573, April 2004*, Copyright 2006 American College of Sports Medicine

166. Weller, Ellen; Bachert, Peter; Meinck, Hans-Michael; Friedmann, Bridgit; Bartsch, Peter; Mairbaurl, Heimo. Lack of Effect of Oral Mg-Supplementation on Mg in Serum, Blood Cells, and Calf Muscle. *Medicine and Science in Sports and Exercise: Volume 30(11) November 1998 pp. 1584-1591 pp. 1584-1591*, Copyright 2006 American College of Sports Medicine

167. Ralph S. Welsh, J. Mark Davis, Jean R. Burke, and Harriet G. Williams. Carbohydrates and Physical/Mental Performance During Intermittent Exercise to Fatigue. *Medicine and Science in*

Sports and Exercise: Volume 34(4) April 2002 pp. 723-731, Copyright 2006 American College of Sports Medicine

168. Wickel, Eric E.; Eisenmann, Joey C.; Welk, Gregory J. Adolescent Aerobic Fitness and Adult Cardiovascular Disease Risk Factors: The Aerobics Center Longitudinal Study. *Medicine and Science in Sports and Exercise: Volume 30(5) Supplement May 1998 p. 218,* Copyright 2006 American College of Sports Medicine

169. Nathan Wilder, Roger Gilders, Frederick Hagerman, and Richard G. Deivert. The Effects of a 10-Week, Periodized, Off-Season Resistance-Training Program and Creatine Supplementation Among Collegiate Football Players. *J. Strength Cond. Res.,* 2002, 16(3), 343-352, Copyright 2002 National Strength and Conditioning Association

170. Wingo, Jonathan; Lafrenze, Andrew; Stueck, Matt, Cureton, Kirk. Effects of Cardiovascular Drift on Maximal Oxygen Uptake: Influence of Hydration. *Medicine and Science in Sports and Exercise: Volume 36(5) Supplement May 2004 p. S331,* Copyright 2006 American College of Sports Medicine

171. Holly R. Wyatt, John C. Peters, George W. Reed, Mary Barry, and James O. Hill. A Colorado Statewide Survey of Walking and Its Relation to Excessive Weight. *Medicine and Science in Sports and Exercise: Volume 37(5) May 2005 p. 724-730,* Copyright 2006 American College of Sports Medicine

172. Judy Kruger, Deborah A. Galuska, Mary K. Serdula, and Harold W. Kohl III. Physical Activity Profiles of U.S. Adults Trying to Lose Weight: NHIS 1998. *Medicine and Science in Sports and Exercise: Volume 37(3) 2005 p. 364-368,* Copyright 2006 American College of Sports Medicine

173. American College of Sports Medicine. Position Stand - The Use of Alcohol in Sports. *Medicine and Science in Sports and Exercise,*

Volume 14(6), Copyright 2006 American College of Sports Medicine

174. Brian M. Peeters, Christopher D. Lantz, and Jerry L. Mayhew. Effect of Oral Creatine Monohydrate and Creatine Phosphate Supplementation on Maximal Strength Indices, Body Composition, and Blood Pressure. . *J. Strength Cond. Res.*, 1999, 13(1), 3-9, Copyright 1999 National Strength and Conditioning Association

Bibliography: Section 2 – Chapter 3, 4 & 5

1. Abt, John; Brick, Matthew; Smoglia, James; Jolly John; Lephart, Scott FACSM; Fu, Freddie. Alterations in Cycling Mechanics Resulting from Core Fatigue: 620 Board #212 2:00pm – 3:30 PM. *Medicine and Science in Sports and Exercise: Volume 37(5) May 2005 p S121-S122*, Copyright 2007 American College of Sports Medicine

2. Thomas R. Baechle, Roger W. Earle. Essentials of Strength Training and Conditioning - 2nd Edition. Copyright 2000, 1994 National Strength and Condition Association

3. Jeffrey A. Bauer, Andrew Fry, and Cory Carter. The Use of Lumbar-Supporting Weight Belts While Performing Squats: Erector Spinae Electromyographic Activity. *J. Strength Cond. Res. 13(4), 384-388 1999*, Copyright 1999 National Strength and Conditioning Association

4. David M. Bazett-Jones, Jason B. Winchester, Jeffrey M. McBride. Effect of Potentiation and Stretching on Maximal Force, Rate of Force Development, and Range of Motion. *J. Strength Con. Res.*

19(2), 421-426, Copyright National Strength and Conditioning Association 2005

5.   David G. Behm. Neuromuscular Implications and Applications of Resistance Training. *J. Strength Cond. Res. 9(4), 264-274.* Copyright 1995, National Strength and Conditioning Association

6.   David G. Behm, Kenneth Anderson, and Robert S. Curnew. Muscle Force and Activation under Stable and Unstable Conditions. *J Strength Cond. Res. 16(3), 416-422. 2002,* Copyright 2002 National Strength and Conditioning Association

7.   Darren G. Burke, Christopher J. Culligan, and Laurence E. Holt. The Theoretical Basis of Proprioceptive Neuromuscular Facilitation. *J. Strength Cond. Res. 14(4), 496-500,* Copyright 2000 National Strength and Conditioning Association

8.   David G. Behm, Allison M. Leonard, Warren B. Young, W. Andrew C. Bonsey, and Scott N MacKinnon. Trunk Muscle Electromyographic Activity with Unstable and Unilateral Exercise. *J. Strength Cond. Res. 19(1), 193-201,* Copyright 2005 National Strength and Conditioning Association

9.   Butcher, S. J.; Craven, B. R.; Sprinings, E. J. C.; Chilibeck, P.D.; Spink, K.S.. Influence of Trunk Stability and Leg Strength Training on Vertical Take-Off Velocity in Athletes. *Medicine and Science in Sports and Exercise: Volume 33(5) Supplement 1 May 2001 p S158,* Copyright 2007 American College of Sports Medicine

10.   Michael A. Clark, Rodney J. Corn.   NASM OPT Optimum Performance Training for the Fitness Professional, 2nd Edition. Copyright 2001 National Academy of Sports Medicine.

11.   Kathryn M. Clark, Laurence E. Holt, and Joy Sinyard. Electromyographic Comparison of the Upper and Lower Rectus Abdominis during Abdominal Activities. *J. Strength Cond.*

Research. 17(3), 475-483. Copyright 2002 National Strength and Conditioning Association

12. 12. Rodney Corn. Putting the Maximus Back in Your Gluteus: Common Causes of Disruption in Neuromuscular Efficiency. Copyright 2002, National Academy of Sports Medicine.

13. Ludmila M. Cosio-Lima, Katy L Reynolds, Christa Winter, Vincent Paolone, and Margaret T. Jones. Effects of Physioball and Conventional Floor Exercises on Early Phase Adaptations in Back and Abdominal Core Stability and Balance in Women. *J. Strength Cond. Res. 17(4), 721-725.* Copyright 2003 National Strength and Conditioning Association

14. Michael R. Deschenes, Carl M Maresh, and William J. Kraemer. The Neuromuscular Junction: Structure, Function, and its Role in the Excitation of Muscle. *J. Strength Cond. Res. 8(2), 103-109* Copyright 1994, National Strength and Conditioning Association

15. Dickenson, E.L.; Crock D. D.; Holbein-Jenny, M. A.. The Isokinetic Strength Training Effect of the Torso Track II versus the Standard Trunk Curl. *Medicine and Science in Sports and Exercise: Volume 34(5) Supplement 1 May 2002 pp S91,* Copyright 2007 American College of Sports Medicine

16. Tammy K. Evetovich, Terry J. Housh, Dona J. Housh, Glen O. Johnson, Douglas B. Smith, and Kyle T. Ebersole. The Effect of Concentric Isokinetic Strength Training, of the Quadriceps Femoris on Electromyography and Muscle Strength in the Trained and Untrained Limb. *J. Strength Cond. Res. 15(4), 439-445,* Copyright National Strength & Conditioning Association 2001

17. Haight, Shara M.; Parr, Richard B. FACSM; Hornak, James E. Effects of Weight Loss on Abdominal Fat Stores in Overweight and Obese Females: 1591 Board #46 11:00am – 12:30 PM 11. *Medicine and*

Science in Sports and Exercise: Volume 37(5) Supplement May 2005 pp S304, Copyright 2007 American College of Sports Medicine

18. Susan J. Hall, Jurip Lee and Terry M. Wood. Evaluation of Selected Sit-up Variations for the Individual with Low Back Pain. *J. of Applied Sports Sci. Research, Volume 4, Number 2, 1990*

19. Tina L. Hayter, Jeff S. Coombers, Wade L. Knez, and Tania L. Brancato. Effects of Electrical Muscle Stimulation on Oxygen Consumption. *J. Strength Cond. Res. 19(1), 98-101.* Copyright 2005 National Strength and Conditioning Association

20. Karl M. Herman and William S. Barnes. Effects of Eccentric Exercise on Trunk Extensor Torque and Lumbar Paraspinal EMG. *Medicine and Science in Sports and Exercise: Volume 33(6) June 2001 pp 971-977,* Copyright 2007 American College of Sports Medicine

21. Hongtao, Ma; Bai, Liu; Yanchun, Yuan. The Study of Methods of Functional Core Stability for Gymnastics Training. *Medicine and Science in Sports and Exercise: Volume 34(5) Supplement 1 May 2002 p 51,* Copyright 2007 American College of Sports Medicine

22. Edward T. Howley, B. Don Franks. Health Fitness Instructors Handbook - 3rd Edition. Human Kinetics, Copyright 1997, 1992, 1986 by Edward T. Howley and B. Don Franks

23. Hunter, Gary R.; Bryan, David R.; Wetzstein, Carla J.; Zuckerman, Paul A.; Bamman, Marcas M.. Resistance Training and Intra-Abdominal Adipose Tissue in Older Men and Women. *Medicine and Science in Sports and Exercise: Volume 34(6) June 2002 pp 1023-1028,* Copyright 2007 American College of Sports Medicine

24. Sandra K. Hunter; Jaques Duchateau; Roger M. Enoka. Reflex Activity and Task Failure. *Exerc. Sport Sci. Rev. 32(2):44-49, 2004.* Copyright 2004 American College of Sports Medicine

25. Kazunori Iwai, Koichi Nakazato, Kazunori Irie, Hideo Fujimoto, and Hiroyuki Nakajima. Trunk Muscle Strength and Disability Level of Low Back Pain in Collegiate Wrestlers. *Medicine and Science in Sports and Exercise: Volume 36(8) 2004 pp 1296-1300,* Copyright 2007 American College of Sports Medicine

26. John M. Jackic, Kristine Clark, Ellen Coleman, Joseph E. Donnely, John Foreyt, Edward Melenson, Jeff Volek, and Stella L. Volpe.. Position Stand: Appropriate Intervention Strategies for Weight Loss and Prevention of Weight Regain for Adults. *Medicine & Science in Sports & Exercise 0195-9131/01/3312-2145* Copyright 2001 American College of Sports Medicine

27. Gregor Lattier, Guillaume Y. Millet, Nicola A. Maffiuletti, Nicholas Babualt, and Romuald Lepers. Neuromuscular Differences between Endurance-Trained, Power-Trained and Sedentary Subjects. *J Strength Cond. Res. 17(3), 514-521* Copyright 2003, National Strength and Conditioning Association

28. Darin T. Leetun, Mary Lloyd Ireland, John D. Willson, Bryon T. Ballantyne, and Irene McClay Davis. Core Stability Measures as Risk Factors for Lower Extremity Injury in Athletes. *Medicine and Science in Sports and Exercise: Volume 36(6) June 2004 pp 926-934,* Copyright 2007 American College of Sports Medicine

29. Jeremy Maynard and William P. Ebben. The Effects of Antagonist Prefatigue on Agonist Torque and Electromyography. *J Strength Cond. Res. 17(3), 469-474* Copyright 2003 National Strength and Conditioning Association

30. Melissa J. Mayo, Justin R. Grantham, and Govindasamy Balasekaren. Exercise-Induced Weight Loss Preferentially Reduces Abdominal Fat. *Medicine and Science in Sports and Exercise: Volume 35(2) February 2003 pp 207-213,* Copyright 2006 American College of Sports Medicine

31. Joseph K.-F. NG, Vaughan Kippers, Mohamad Parnianpour, and Carolyn A. Richardson. EMG Activity Normalization for Trunk Muscles in Subjects With and Without Back Pain. *Medicine and Science in Sports and Exercise: Volume 34(7) 2002 pp 1082-1086,* Copyright 2007 American College of Sports Medicine

32. Nindl, Bradley C.; Freidl, Karl E.; Marchitelli, Louis J.; Shippee, Ronald L.; Thomas, Cecilia D.: Patton, John F.. Regional Fat Placement in Physically Fit Males and Changes with Weight Loss. *Medicine and Science in Sports and Exercise: Volume 28(7) July 1996 pp. 786-793,* Copyright 2006 American College of Sports Medicine

33. 33. Jeremy Pick and M. Daniel Becque. The Relationship between Training Status and the Intensity on Muscle Activation and Relative Submaximal Lifting Capacity during the Back Squat. *J. Strength and Cond. Res. 14(2), 175-182 Copyright 2000,* National Strength and Conditioning Association

34. John P. Porcari, Karen Palmer McClean, Carl Foster, Thomas Kernozek, Ben Crenshaw, and Chad Swanson. Effects of Electrical Muscle Stimulation on Body Composition, Muscle Strength, and Physical Appearance. *J. Strength Cond. Res. 16(2), 165-172.* Copyright 2002 National Strength and Conditioning Association

35. Mike Ross, Susan J. Hall, Nick Briet, and Sam Britten. Effect of a Lumbar Support Device on Muscle Activity during Abdominal Exercises. *J. Strength Cond. Res. 7(4), 219-223,* Copyright 1993 National Strength and Conditioning Association

36. Christine L. Ruther, Catherine L. Golden, Robert T. Harris, and Gary A. Dudley. Hypertrophy, Resistance Training and the Nature of Skeletal Muscle Activation. *J. Strength Cond. Res. 9(3), 155-159.* Copyright 1995 National Strength and Conditioning Association

37. Ross, Robert; Janssen, Ian.   Is Abdominal Fat Preferentially Reduced in Response to Exercise-Induced Weight Loss? *Medicine and Science in Sports and Exercise: Volume 31(11) Supplement 1 November 1999 p. S568,* Copyright 2006 American College of Sports Medicine

38. William A. Sands and Jeni R. McNeal. A Kinematic Comparison of Four Abdominal Training Devices and a Traditional Abdominal Crunch. *J. Strength Cond. Res. 16(1), 135-141.* Copyright 2002 National Strength and Conditioning Association

39. Roberto Simao, Paulo de Tarso Veras Farinatti, Marcos Doederlein Polito, Alex Souto Major, and Steven J. Fleck. Influence of Exercise Order on the Number of Repetitions Performed and Perceived Exertion During Resistance Exercises. *J. Strength Cond. Res.* 19(1), 152-156. Copyright 2005 National Strength and Conditioning Association

40. Eric Sternlicht, Stuart G. Rugg, Matt D. Bernstein, and Scott D. Armstrong. Electromyographical Analysis and Comparison of Selected Abdominal Training Devices with a Traditional Crunch. *J. Strength Cond. Res. 19(1), 157-162.* Copyright 2005 National Strength and Conditioning Association

41. Eric Sternlicht and Stuart Rugg. Electromyographic Analysis of Abdominal Muscle Activity Using Portable Abdominal Exercise Devices and a Traditional Crunch. *J. Strength Cond. Res. 17(3), 463-468.* Copyright 2003 National Strength and Conditioning Association.

42. Thompson, Christian; Blackwell, John; Kepesidis, Ioannis; Myers-Cobb, Karen. Effects of Core Stabilization on Fitness, Swing Speed, and Weight Transfer in Older Male Golfers. *Medicine and Science in Sports and Exercise: Volume 36(5) May 2004 p S204,* Copyright 2007 American College of Sports Medicine

43. Susan B. Votruba, Richard L. Atkinson, Matt D. Hirvonen, and Dale A. Schoeller. Prior Exercise Increases Subsequent Utilization of Dietary Fat. *Medicine and Science in Sports and Exercise: Volume 34(11) November 2002 pp 1757-1765*, Copyright 2006 American College of Sports Medicine

44. Lawrence W. Weiss, Larry E. Wood, Andrew C. Fry, Richard B. Kreider, George E. Relyea, Daryl B. Bullen, and Pamela D. Grindstaff. Strength/Power Augmentation Subsequent to Short-Term Training Abstinence. *J. Strength Cond. Res. 18(4), 765-770.* Copyright 2004 National Strength and Conditioning Association

45. William C. Whiting, Stuart Rugg, Andre Coleman, and William J. Vincent. Muscle Activity during Sit-ups Using Abdominal Exercise Devices. *J. Strength Cond. Res. 13(4), 339-345.* Copyright 1999 National Strength and Conditioning Association

46. Glenn N. Williams; Peter J. Barrance; Lynn Snyder-Mackler; Thomas S. Buchanan. Altered Quadriceps Control in People With Anterior Cruciate Ligament Deficiency. *From Medicine & Science in Sports & Exercise http://www.medscape.com/viewarticle/482930*

47. John D. Willson, Mary Lloyd Ireland, and Irene Davis. Core Strength and Lower Extremity Alignment during Single Leg Squats. Medicine and Science in Sports and Exercise: *Volume 38(5) 2006 pp 945-952,* Copyright 2007 American College of Sports Medicine

48. Jack H. Wilmore, David L. Costill. Physiology of Sport and Exercise – Third Edition, *Copyright 2004 Jack H Wilmore and David L. Costill. Publisher Human Kinetics.*

49. You, Tongjian; Lyles, Mary F.; Nicklas, Barbara J.. Addition of Exercise Training To Dietary Weight Loss Reduces Abdominal, But Not Gluteal Adipocyte Size: 751 9:00 AM – 9:15AM. *Medicine and*

Science in Sports and Exercise: Volume 37(5) Supplement May 2005 pp S137, Copyright 2007 American College of Sports Medicine

50. Raymond C. Browning, Jesse R. Modica, Rodger Kram, and Ambarish Goswami. The Effects of Adding Mass to the Legs on the Energetics and Biomechanics of Walking. *Medicine and Science in Sports and Exercise: Volume 39(3) March 2007 pp 515-525,* Copyright 2007 American College of Sports Medicine

51. Carpenter DM, Graves JE, Pollock ML, Leggett SH, Foster D, Holmes B, Fulton MN. Effect of 12 and20 weeks of resistance training on lumbar extension torque production. *Phys Ther.* 1991 Aug; 71(8):580-8.

52. DeMichele PL, Pollock ML, Graves JE, Foster DN, Carpenter D, Garzarella L, Brechue W, Fulton M. Isometric torso rotation strength: effect of training frequency on its development. *Arch Phys Med Rehabil.* 1997 Jan;78(1);64-69

Bibliography:
Section 3: Chapter 6

1. ACSM News Release: ACSM Releases New Position Stand on Resistance Training Progression, *News Release:* Director, Gail N. Hunt.
http://www.acsm.org/publications/newsreleases2002/ResTrainProg021002.htm

2. American College of Sports Medicine. ACSM's Guidelines for Exercise Testing and Prescription, Sixth Edition; Senior Editor Barry A. Franklin, Associate Editor Mitchell H. Whaley and Edward T. Howley; Authors Gary J. Dalady.... [et. al.] Copyright 2001 American College of Sports Medicine

3. ACSM News Release: Physical Activity Reduces Breast Cancer Risk: Duration More Important Than Intensity, *News Release: Director*, Gail N. Hunt.
http://www.acsm.org/publications/newsreleases2001/risk.htm

4. Juha P. Ahtiainen, Arto Pakarinen, Markku Alen, William J. Lraemer, and Keijo Hakkinen. Short vs. Long Rest Period Between the Sets in Hypertrophic Resistance Training: Influence on Muscle Strength, Size, and Hormonal Adaptations in Trained Men. *J. Strength Cond. Res.* 19(3), 572-582, Copyright 20015National Strength & Conditioning Association

5. Thomas R. Baechle, Roger W. Earle. Essentials of Strength Training and Conditioning - 2nd Edition. Copyright 2000, 1994 National Strength and Condition Association

6. David G. Behm, Gregory Reardon, James Fitzgerald, and Eric Drinkwater. The Effect of 5,10, and 20 Repetition Maximums on the Recovery of Voluntary and Evoked Contractile Properties. *J. Strength Cond. Res.* 16(2), 209-218, Copyright 2002 National Strength & Conditioning Association

7. David G. Behm, Kellie M. Baker, Robert Kelland, and Jason Lomond. The Effect of Muscle Damage on Strength and Fatigue Deficits. *J. Strength Cond. Res.* 15(2), 225-263, Copyright 2001 National Strength & Conditioning Association

8. Holly M. Bilcheck, Carl M. Maresh, William J. Kraener. Muscular Fatigue: A Brief Overview. *J. Strength Cond. Res.* 14(6) 9-13, Copyright 1992 National Strength & Conditioning Association

9. Kerry J. Bosher, Jeffrey A. Pottieger, Chris Gennings, Paul E. Luebbers, Keith A. Shannon, Robynn M. Shannon. Effects of different macronutrient consumption following a resistance-training session on fat and carbohydrate metabolism. *J. Strength*

Cond. Res. 18(2) 212-219, Copyright 1992 National Strength & Conditioning Association

10. Jenn V. Brazell-Roberts and Luke E. Thomas. Effects of Weight Training Frequency on the Self-concept of College Females. *J. of Applied Sports Science Research* 3(2) 40-43, Copyright 1989

11. Bruan WA, Hawthorne WE, Markofski MN. Acute EPOC response in women to circuit training and treadmill exercise of matched oxygen consumption. *Eur J Appl Physiol.* 2005 Aug:94(5-6):500-4 Epub 2005 Jun 8.

12. Carpenter DM, Graves JE, Pollock ML, Leggett SH, Foster D, Holmes B, Fulton MN. Effect of 12 and 20 weeks of resistance training on lumbar extension torque production. *Phys Ther.* 1991 Aug; 71(8):580-8.

13. Michael A. Clark, Rodney J. Corn. NASM OPT Optimum Performance Training for the Fitness Professional, 2nd Edition. Copyright 2001, National Academy of Sports Medicine.

14. DeMichele PL, Pollock ML, Graves JE, Foster DN, Carpenter D, Garzarella L, Brechue W, Fulton M. Isometric torso rotation strength: effect of training frequency on its development. *Arch Phys Med Rehabil.* 1997 Jan;78(1);64-69

15. Coop DeRenne, Ronald K Hetzler, Barton P. Buxton, Kwok W. Ho. Effects of Training Frequency on Strength Maintenance in Pubescent Baseball Players. *J. Strength Cond. Res.* 10(1), 8-14, Copyright 1996 National Strength & Conditioning Association

16. Micah J. Drummond, Pat R. Vehrs, G. Bruce Schaalje, and Allen C. Parcell. Aerobic and Resistance Exercise Sequence affects Excess Post Exercise Oxygen Consumption. *J. Strength Cond. Res.* 19(2), 332-337, Copyright 2005 National Strength & Conditioning Association

17. Fatouros IG, Taxildaris K, Tokmakidis SP, Kalapotharokos V, Aggelousis N, Athanasopoulus S, Zeeris I, Katrabasas I. The effects of strength training, cardiovascular training and their combination on flexibility of inactive older adults. *Int J Sports Med* 2002 Feb;23(2))112-9

18. Ferrara CM, McCrone SH, Brendle D, Ryan AS, Goldberg AP. Metabolic effects of the addition of resistive to aerobic exercise in older men. *Int J Sport Nutr Exerc Metab.* 2004 Feb;14(1):73-80.

19. Daniel A. Galvao and Dennis R. Taafe. Single- vs. Multiple-Set Resistance Training: Recent Development in the Controversy. *J. Strength Cond. Res.* 18(3), 660-667, Copyright 2005 National Strength & Conditioning Association

20. Randall E. Gearhart, Jr. Fredric L. Goss, Kristen M. Lagally, John M Jakicic, Jere Gallagher, Kara I. Gallagher, and Robert J. Robertson. Rating of Perceived Exertion in Active Muscle During High-Intensity and Low-Intensity Resistance Exercise. *J. Strength Cond. Res.* 16(1), 87-91, Copyright 2002 National Strength & Conditioning Association

21. Girouard CK, Hurley BF. Does strength training inhibit gains in range of motion from flexibility training in older adults. *Med Sci Sports Exerc.* 1995 Oct;27(10):1444-9

22. Juan J. Gonzalez-Badillo, Esteban M. Gorostiaga, Raul Arellano, and Mikel Izquierdo. Moderate Resistance Training Volume Produces More Favorable Strength Gains Than High or Low Volumes During a Short-Term Training Cycle. *J. Strength Cond. Res.* 19(3), 689-697, Copyright 2005 National Strength & Conditioning Association

23. Kazushige Goto, Masanari Nagasawa, Osuma Yanagisawa, Tomohiro Kizuka, Naokata Ishii, and Kaoru Takamatsu. Muscular Adaptations to a Combinations of High- and Low-Intensity

Resistance Exercises. *J. Strength Cond. Res.* 18(4), 730-737, Copyright 2004 National Strength & Conditioning Association

24. Graves JE, Pollock ML, Leggett SH, Carpenter DM, Fix CK, Fulton MN. Limited range-of-motion lumbar extension strength training. *Med Sci Sports Exerc.* 1992 Jan;24(1):128-33

25. G. Gregory Haff. Fitness Frontlines. Fitness Frontlines: Combination Training Results in Significant Decreases in Abdominal Fat Mass. *NSCA's Performance Training Journal* 3(6) 15 Copyright 2005 National Strength and Conditioning Journal www.nsca-lift.org/perform

26. Jay R. Hoffman, William J. Kraemer, Andrew C. Fry, Michael Dechenes, and Michael Kemp. The Effects of Self-Selection for Frequency of Training in a Winter Conditioning Program for Football. *Journal of Applied Sports Science and Research Cond. Res.* 3(4),76-82 , 1990

27. Hakkinen K, Alen M, Kraemer WJ, Gorostiaga E, Izquierdo M, Rusko H, Mikkola J, Hakkinen A, Valkeinen H, Kaarakainen E, Romu S, Erola V, Ahtiainen J, Paavolainen L. Neuromuscular adaptations during concurrent strength and endurance training versus strength training. *Eur J Appl Physiol.* 2003 Mar;89(1):42-52 Epub 2002 Dec. 14

28. Chad Harris, Mark A. DeBeliso, Terry A. Spitzer-Gibson, and Kent J. Adams. The Effect of Resistance-Training Intensity on Strength-Gain Response in the Older Adult. *J. Strength Cond. Res.* 18(4) 833-838, Copyright 2004 National Strength & Conditioning Association

29. Edward T. Howley, B. Don Franks. Health Fitness Instructors Handbook - 3rd Edition. Human Kinetics, Copyright 1997, 1992, 1986 by Edward T. Howley and B. Don Franks

30. Joe Kang, Jay R. Hoffman, Joohee Im, Barry A. Spiering, Nicholas A. Ratamess, Kenneth W. Rundell, Shoko Nioka, Joshua Cooper, and Britton Chance. Evaluation of Physiological Responses During Recovery Following Three Resistance Exercise Programs. *J. Strength Cond. Res.* 19(2), 305-309 Copyright 2005 National Strength & Conditioning Association

31. Naoki Kawamori and G. Gregory Haff. The Optimal Training Load for the Development of Muscular Power. *J. Strength Cond. Res.* 18(3), 675-684 Copyright 2004 National Strength & Conditioning Association

32. Kraemer WJ, Vescovi JD, Volek JS, Nindi BC, Newton RU, Patton JF, Dziados JE, French DN Hakkinen K. Effects of concurrent resistance and aerobic training on load-bearing performance and the Army Physical fitness test. *Mil Med.* 2004 Dec;169(12):994-9

33. Wolfgang K. Kremmler, Dirk Lauber, Klaus Engelke, and Juergen Weineck. Effects of Single- vs. Multiple-set Resistance Training on Maximum Strength and Body Composition in Trained Postmenopausal Women. *J. Strength Cond. Res.* 18(2), 359-364, Copyright 2004 National Strength & Conditioning Association

34. Kristen M. Lagally, Steven T. McCaw, Geoff T. Young, Heather C. Medema, and David Q Thomas. Rating of Perceived Exertion and Muscle Activity During the Bench Press Exercise in Recreational and Novice Lifters. *J. Strength Cond. Res.* 18(3), 660-667, Copyright 2005 National Strength & Conditioning Association

35. Andrew Lee, Bruce W. Craig, Jeff Lucas, Roberta Pohlman, and Herbert Stelling. The Effect of Endurance Training, Weight Training and A Combination of Endurance and Weight Training Upon the Blood Lipid Profile of Young Male Subjects. *J. Strength Cond. Res.* 4(3), 68-75, Copyright 1990 National Strength & Conditioning Association

36. Lewis DA, Kamon E, Hodgson JL. Physiological differences between genders. Implications for sports conditioning. *Sports Med.* 1986 Sep-Oct;3(5):357-69.

37. S. P.Magnusson, P. Aagaard, E.B. Simonsen, F. Bojsen-Moller. Passive tensile stress and energy of the human hamstring muscles in vivo. *Scandinavian Journal of Medicine & Science in Sports* 10(6) 351 - December 2000

38. C. Dwayne Massey, John Vincent, Mark Maneval, Melissa Moore, and J.T. Johnson. An Analysis of Full Range of Motion vs. Partial Range of Motion Training in the Development of Strength in Untrained Men. *J. Strength Cond. Res.* 18(3), 518-521 Copyright 2004 National Strength & Conditioning Association

39. C. Dwayne Massey, John Vincent, Mark Maneval, Melissa Moore, and J.T. Johnson. Influence of Range of Motion in Resistance Training in Women: Early Phase Adaptations. *J. Strength Cond. Res.* 19(2), 409-411 Copyright 2005 National Strength & Conditioning Association

40. McCarrick MJ, Kemp JG. The effect of strength training and reduced training on rotator cuff musculature. *Clin. Biomech* (Bristol, Avon). 2000; 15 Suppl 1:S42-5

41. John R McLester, Jr., P. Bishop, and M.E. Guilliams. Comparison of 1 Day and 3 Days Per Week of Equal-Volume Resistance Training in Experienced Subjects. *J. Strength Cond. Res.* 14(3) 273-281, Copyright 2000 National Strength & Conditioning Association

42. John R. McLester, Phillip A. Bishop, Joe Smith, Lana Wyers, Barry Dale, Joseph Kozusko, Mark Richardson, Michael E. Nevett, and Richard Lomax. A Series of Studies---A Practical Protocol for Testing Muscular Endurance Recovery. *J. Strength Cond. Res.* 17(2), 259-273, Copyright 2003 National Strength & Conditioning Association

43. Edward L. Melanson, Teresa A. Sharp, Helen M. Seagle, William T. Donahoo, Gary K. Grunwald, John C. Peters, Jere T. Hamilton, James O. Hill. Twenty-Four-Hour Metabolic Responses to Resistance Exercise in Women. *J. Strength Cond. Res.* 19)1), 61-66 Copyright 2005 National Strength & Conditioning Association

44. Morrissey MC, Harman EA, Johnson MJ. Resistance training modes: specificity and effectiveness. Med Sci Sports Exerc. 1995 May;27(5):648-660

45. NSCA Position Statement Briefs: Basic Guidelines for the Resistance Training of Athletes http://nsca-lift.org/Publications/posstatements.shtml

46. Vassilios Paschalis, Yiannis Koutedakis, Athanasios Z. Jamurtas, Vassilis Mougios, and Vasssilios Baltzopoulos. Equal Volumes of High and Low Intensity of Eccentric Exercise in Relation to Muscle Damage and Performance. *J. Strength Cond. Res.* 19(1), 184-188, Copyright 2005 National Strength & Conditioning Association

47. Goran Paulsen, Dag Myklestad, and Truls Raastad. The Influence of Volume of Exercise on Early Adaptations to Strength Training. *J. Strength Cond. Res.* 17(1), 115-120, Copyright 2003 National Strength & Conditioning Association

48. Mark D. Peterson, Matthew R. Rhea, and Brent A. Alvar. Maximizing Strength Development in Athletes: A Meta-Analysis to Determine Dose Response Relationship. *J. Strength Cond. Res.* 18(2), 377-382, Copyright 2004 National Strength & Conditioning Association

49. Danny M. Pincivero, Scott M. Lephart, and Raj G. Karunakura. Effects of Intrasession Rest Interval on Strength Recovery and Reliability During High Intensity Exercise. *J. Strength Cond. Res.*

12(3), 152-156, Copyright 1998 National Strength & Conditioning Association

50. Pollock ML, Graves JE, Bamman MM, Leggett SH, Carpenter DM, Carr C, Cirulli J, Matkozich J, Fulton M. Frequency and volume of resistance training: effect on cervical extension strength. *Arch Phys Med Rehabil.* 1993 Oct;74(10);1080-6

51. Teemu Pullinen, Antii Merq, Pirkko Huttunen, Arto Pakarinin, and Paavo V. Komi. Hormonal Responses to Resistance Exercise Perforrned Under the Influence of Delayed Onset Muscle Soreness. *J. Strength Cond. Res.* 16 (3) 383-389, Copyright 2004 National Strength & Conditioning Association

52. Rhea, Alvar, Ball, Burkett. Three Sets of Weight Training Superior to 1 Set With Equal Intensity for Eliciting Strength. *J. Strength Cond. Res.* 16(4), 525-529, Copyright 2002 National Strength & Conditioning Association

53. E. Todd Schroeder, Steven A. Hawkins, and S. Victoria Jaque. Musculoskeletal Adaptations to 16 Weeks of Eccentric Progressive Resistance Training in Young Women. *J. Strength Cond. Res.* 18(2), 227-235. Copyright 2004 National Strength and Conditioning Association

54. Joseph F. Signorile, Brad Weber, Brad Roll, John F. Caruso, Ilka Lowensteyn, and Arlette C. Perry. An Electromyographical Comparison of the squat and knee Extension Exercises. *J. Strength Cond. Res.* 8(3), 178-183, Copyright 1994 National Strength & Conditioning Association

55. Roberto Simao, Paulo de Tarso Veras Farinatti, Marcos Doederlein Polito, Alex Souto Major, and Steven J. Fleck. Influence of Exercise Order on the Number of Repetitions Performed and Perceived Exertion During Resistance Exercises. *J. Strength Cond. Res.* 19(1),

152-156. Copyright 2005 National Strength and Conditioning Association

56. Sorichter, Stephan; Mair, Johannes; Koller, Arnold; Secnik, Peter; Parrak, Vojtech; Haid, Christian; Muller, Erich; Puscendorf, Bernd. Muscular adaptation and strength during the early phase of eccentric training: influence of the training frequency. *Medicine & Science in Sports and Exercise.* 29(12):1646-1652

57. Ben C. Sporer and Howard A. Wenger. Effects of Aerobic Exercise on Strength Performance Following Various Periods of Recovery. *J. Strength Cond. Res.* 17(4), 638-644. Copyright 2005 National Strength and Conditioning Association

58. Taffe DR, Duret C, Wheeler S, Marcus R. Ounce-weekly resistance exercise improves muscle strength and neuromuscular performance in older adults. *J. Am Geriatr. Soc.* 1999 Oct;47(10):1208-14

59. Takeshima N, Rogers ME Islam MN, Yamauchi T, Watanabe E, Okada A. Effect of concurrent aerobic and resistance circuit exercise training on fitness in older adults. *Eur J Appl Physiol.* 2004 Oct;93(1-2):173-82. Epub 2004 Aug 4

60. Benedict Tan. Manipulating Resistance Training Program Variables to Optimize Strength in Men: A Review. *J. Strength Cond. Res.* 13(3), 289-304, Copyright 1999 National Strength & Conditioning Association

61. Tucci JT, Carpenter DM, Pollock ML, Graves JE, Leggett SH. Effect of Reduced frequency of training and detraining on lumbar extension exercise. *Spine.* 1992 Dec;17(12);1497-501

62. Lawrence W. Weiss, Larry E. Wood, Andrew C. Fry, Richard B. Kreider, George E. Relyea, Daryl B. Bullen, and Pamela D. Grindstaff. Strength/Power Augmentation Subsequent to Short-

Term Training Abstinence. *J. Strength Cond. Res.* 18(4) 765-770, Copyright 2004 National Strength & Conditioning Association

63. Wiemann K, Hahn K. Influences of strength, stretching and circulatory exercises on flexibility parameters of the human hamstrings. *Int J Sports Med.* 1997 Jul;18(5):340-6

64. Brian L/ Wolfe, Linda M. Lemura, and Phillip J. Cole. Quantitative Analysis of Single- vs. Multiple-Set Programs in Resistance Training. *J. Strength Cond. Res.* 18(1), 35-47, Copyright 2004 National Strength & Conditioning Association

65. ACSM Position Stand: Exercise and Hypertension. *Medicine & Science in Sports and Exercise.* Copyright 1993 American College of sports Medicine

66. 66. Stephen C. Glass, Douglas R. Stanton. *Self-Selected Resistance Training Intensity in Novice Weightlifters,* Journal of Strength and Conditioning Research, 2004, 18(2), 324-327 / Copyright 2004 National Strength and Conditioning Association

67. Blundell, John E,; King, Neil A. Physical Activity and Regulation of Food Intake: Current Evidence. *Medicine and Science in Sports and Exercise: Volume 31(11) Supplement 1 November 1999 pp. S573,* Copyright 2006 American College of Sports Medicine

Bibliography:
Section 3: Chapter 7

1. Abe, Takashi; Kawakami, Yasuo; Sugita, Masaaki; Fukunaga, Tetsuo.   Relationships Between Training Frequency and Subcutaneous and Visceral Fat in Women. *Medicine and Science in*

Bibliography

Sports and Exercise: Volume 29(12) p. 1549-1553, 1997, Copyright 2006 American College of Sports Medicine

2. Ainsworth, B. E., Wheeler, F. C.; Huang, Y. Shepard, D. Frequency & Duration of Weekly Physical Activity. *Medicine and Science in Sports and Exercise: Volume 30(5) Supplement May 1998 p. 3*, Copyright 2006 American College of Sports Medicine

3. Aizawa, Kunihiko; Marin, Mauricio; Castro, Isidro Torres; Lawrence, Michele A.; Manley, Jennifer A.; Shoemaker, Kevin J.; Petrella, Robert J. Effects of Lifestyle Modification on Cardiovascular Function in Those at Risk for Cardiovascular Disease: 492 Board #83 2:00 PM - 3:30 PM. *Medicine and Science in Sports and Exercise: Volume 37(5) Supplement May 2005 p. S92*, Copyright 2005 American College of Sports Medicine

4. Albano, C.; Terbizan, D. J.. Heart Rate and RPE Difference Between Aerobic Dance and Cardio-Kickboxing. *Medicine and Science in Sports and Exercise: Volume 33(5) Supplement 1 May 2001 p. S107*, Copyright 2006 American College of Sports

5. Alderman, Brandon L.; Landers, Daniel M. The Influence of Cardiorespiratory Fitness and Hostility on Cardiovascular Reactivity to Mental Stress. *Medicine and Science in Sports and Exercise: Volume 36(5) Supplement May 2004 p. S91*, Copyright 2006 American College of Sports

6. American College of Sports Medicine. ACSM's Guidelines for Exercise Testing and Prescription, Sixth Edition; Senior Editor Barry A. Franklin, Associate Editor Mitchell H. Whaley and Edward T. Howley; Authors Gary J. Dalady.... [et. al.] Copyright 2001 American College of Sports Medicine

7. American College of Sports Medicine. Position Stand - Appropriate Intervention Strategies for Weight Loss and Prevention of Weight Regain for Adults. *Medicine & Science in*

Sports & Exercise Copyright 2001 American College of Sports Medicine

8.   American College of Sports Medicine. Position Stand - Exercise and Type 2 Diabetes. *Medicine & Science in Sports & Exercise* Copyright 2006 American College of Sports Medicine

9.   American College of Sports Medicine. Position Stand - Exercise and Fluid Replacement. *Medicine and Science in Sports and Exercise: Volume 28(1) January 1996,* Copyright 2006 American College of Sports

10. American College of Sports Medicine. Position Stand - Exercise and Hypertension. *Medicine & Science in Sports & Exercise* Copyright 2001 American College of Sports Medicine

11. American College of Sports Medicine. Joint Position Statement-Nutrition and Athletic Performance. *Medicine &Science in Sports and Exercise* Copyright 2000 American College of Sports Medicine.

12. American College of Sports Medicine. Position Stand - Physical Activity and Bone Health. *Medicine & Science in Sports & Exercise* Copyright 2004 American College of Sports Medicine

13. American College of Sports Medicine. Position Stand - The Recommended Quantity and Quality of Exercise for Developing and Maintaining Cardiorespiratory and Muscular Fitness, and Flexibility in Healthy Adults. *Medicine & Science in Sports & Exercise 30(6) June, 1998* Copyright 2006 American College of Sports Medicine

14. Andreacci, Joseph L.; Robertson, Robert J.; Goss Fred L.; Randall, Colby R.; Tessmer Kate A. Frequency of Verbal Encouragement Effects Sub-Maximal Exertional Perceptions During Exercise Testing in Young Adult Swimmers. *Medicine and Science in*

Sports and Exercise: Volume 36(5) Supplement May 2004 p. S133, Copyright 2006 American College of Sports Medicine

15. Ardern, Chris I.; Katzmarzyk, Peter T.; Janssen, Ian; Church, Timothy S.; Blair, Steven N. Adult Treatment Panel III Guidelines and Cardiovascular Disease Mortality: Impact of Cardiorespiratory Fitness. *Medicine and Science in Sports and Exercise: Volume 36(5) Supplement May 2004 p. S135,* Copyright 2006 American College of Sports Medicine

16. Lawrence E. Armstrong, Carl M. Maresh, Micahel Whittlesey, Michael F. Bergeron, Catherine Gabaree, and Jay R. Hoffman. Longitudinal Exercise Heat Tolerance and Running Economy of Collegiate Distance Runners. *J. Strength Cond. Res.* 8(3), 192-197, 1994, Copyright 1994 National Strength and Conditioning Association

17. Todd A. Astorino, Andrew C. Marraco, Sara M. Gross, David L. Johnson, Colleen M. Brazil, Michelette E. Icenhower, & Ryan J. Kneessi. Is Running Performance Enhanced With Creatine Serum Ingestion? *J. Strength Cond. Res.* 19(4), 730-734, 2005, Copyright 2005 National Strength and Conditioning Association

18. Thomas R. Baechle, Roger W. Earle. Essentials of Strength Training and Conditioning - 2nd Edition. Copyright 2000, 1994 National Strength and Condition Association

19. Christos P. Balabinis, Charalampos H. Psarakis, Makkos Moukas, Miltos P. Vissoliou, and Panagiotos K. Behrakis. Early Phase Changes by Concurrent Endurance and Strength Training. *J. Strength Cond. Res. 17(2), 393-401, 2003.* Copyright 2003 National Strength and Conditioning Association

20. Baynard T.; Szymanski, L/; Clara, H Santa; Fernhall, B. Racial Differences in Regional Weight Loss After Exercise Training Does Not Alter Cardiovascular Risk. *Medicine and Science in Sports and*

Exercise: Volume 35(5) Supplement 1 May 2003 p. S374, Copyright 2006 American College of Sports Medicine

21. Craig J. Biwer, Randall L. Jensen, W. Daniel Schmidt, and Phillip B. Watts. The Effect of Creatine on Treadmill Running With High-Intensity Intervals. *J. Strength Cond. Res.* 17(3), 439-445, Copyright 2003 National Strength and Conditioning Association

22. Brandley, D.; Santiago, M.; Oddou, W. Influence of Step Height and Frequency on Cardiac and Metabolic Work During Stairclimbing Ergometry 1231. *Medicine and Science in Sports and Exercise: Volume 28(5) Supplement May 1996 p. 207,* Copyright 2006 American College of Sports

23. Thierry Busso. Variable Dose-Response Relationship Between Exercise Training and Performance. *Medicine and Science in Sports and Exercise: Volume 35(7) p. 1188-1195, 2003* Copyright 2006 American College of Sports Medicine

24. Samuel Case, Thomas Redmond, Scott Currey, Matthew Wachter, and Jerry Resh. The Effects of the Breathe Right Nasal Strip on Interval Running Performance. *J. Strength Cond. Res. 12(1), 30-32, 1998.* Copyright 1998 National Strength and Conditioning Association

25. Yiling J. Cheng, Caroline A. Macera, Timothy S. Church, and Steven N. Blair. Heart Rate Reserve as a Predictor of Cardiovascular and All Cause Mortality in Men. *Medicine and Science in Sports and Exercise: Volume 34(12) p. 1873-1878, 2002* Copyright 2006 American College of Sports Medicine

26. Christou, D. D.; Gates, P.E.; Seals, D. R. Is Fatness or Fitness the Best Predictor of Cardiovascular Disease Risk Profile in Healthy Men? *Medicine and Science in Sports and Exercise: Volume 35(5) Supplement 1 May 2003 p. S67,* Copyright 2006 American College of Sports Medicine

27. Michael A. Clark, Rodney J. Corn.   NASM OPT Optimum Performance Training for the Fitness Professional, 2nd Edition Copyright 2001, National Academy of Sports Medicine.

28. Cox, J.O.; Flohr, J. A.; Saunders, M.J.; Todd, M. K. The Effects of 12 Weeks of Cardioresistance, Resistance, or Cardiovascular Training on Blood Lipids. *Medicine and Science in Sports and Exercise: Volume 33(5) Supplement 1 May 2001 p. S229,* Copyright 2006 American College of Sports Medicine

29. Bruce W. Craig, Jeff Lucas, Roberta, Pohlman, and Herbert Stellin. The Effects of Running, Weightlifting and a Combination of Both on Growth Hormone Release. *Journal of Applied Sports Science Research 3(4) pp. 198-203, 1991*

30. DeSisso, Travis D.; Gerst Jonathan W.; Carnathan, Patrick D.; Kukta,Leslie C.; Skelton, Lauren E.; Bland, Justin R.; Turley, Kenneth R. Effect of Caffeine on Metabolic and Cardiovascular Responses to Submaximal Exercises: Boys Versus Men: 2429 2:00 PM - 2:15 PM *Medicine and Science in Sports and Exercise: Volume 37(5) Supplement May 2005 p. S465,* Copyright 2006 American College of Sports Medicine

31. Dasgupta, Kaberi; Grover, Steven A.; Lowensteyn, Ilka; Chan, Deborah; Rahme, Elham. Relationship between Cardiovascular Fitness and Cardiovascular Risk Among Obese Patients with Type 2 Diabetes. *Medicine and Science in Sports and Exercise: Volume 36(5) Supplement May 2004 p. S141,* Copyright 2006 American College of Sports Medicine

32. Dasgupta, Kaberi; Grover, Steven A.; Lowensteyn, Ilka; Chan, Deborah; DaCosta, Deborah; Yale, Jean-Francois; Iqbal, Sameena; Jimenez, Vania; Rahme, Elham. Supervised Exercise and Diet in Type 2 Diabetes: Impact on Weight and Cardiovascular Risk Factors: 1975 Board #114 3:30 PM - 5:00 PM. *Medicine and Science*

in Sports and Exercise: Volume 37(5) Supplement May 2005 p. S381, Copyright 2006 American College of Sports Medicine

33. Leo J. D'Acquisto, Debra M. D'Acquiso, and Dave Renne. Metabolic and Cardiovascular Responses in Older Women During Shallow-Water Exercise. *J. Strength Cond. Res.* 15(1), 12-19, 2001, Copyright 2001 National Strength and Conditioning Association

34. Glenn E. Duncan, Sierra M. Li, and Xiao-Hua Zhou. Cardiovascular Fitness among U.S Adults NHANES 1999-2000 and 2001-2002. *Medicine and Science in Sports and Exercise: Volume 37(8) 2005 p. 1324-1328,* Copyright 2006 American College of Sports Medicine

35. Dunn, A. L.; Trivedi, M. H.; Kampert, J. B.; O'Neal, H. A.; Clark, C. G. Exercise Dose-Response and The Treatment of Major Depression. *Medicine and Science in Sports and Exercise: Volume 34(5) Supplement 1 May 2002 p. S239,* Copyright 2006 American College of Sports Medicine

36. Andrea L. Dunn, Madhukar H. Trivedi, and Heather A. O'Neal. Physical activity Dose-Response Effects on Outcomes of Depression and Anxiety. *Medicine and Science in Sports and Exercise: Volume 33(6) Suppl. 2001 p. S587-S597,* Copyright 2006 American College of Sports Medicine

37. Conrad P. Earnest, Stacey L. Lancaster, Christopher J. Rasmussen, Chad M. Kerksick, Alejandro Lucia, Michael C. Greenwood, Anthony L. Almada, Patty A. Cowan, and Richard B. Krieder. Low Vs. High Glycemic Index Carbohydrate Gel Ingestion During Simulated 64-KM Cycling Time Trial Performance. *J. Strength Cond. Res.* 18(3), 466-472, Copyright 2004 National Strength and Conditioning Association

38. William P. Ebben, Alan G. Kindler, Kerri A Chirdon, Nina C. Jenkins. The Effect of High -Load vs. High -Repetition Training on Endurance Performance. *J. Strength Cond. Res. 18(3), 513-517, 2004.* Copyright 2004 National Strength and Conditioning Association

39. Eisenmann, Joey, C.; Welk, Gregory J.; Wickel, Eric E.; Blair, Steven N. Cardiorespiratory Fitness, Body Mass Index and Cardiovascular Disease Risk Factors Among Children and Adolescents: The Aerobics Center Longitudinal Study: 1503 9:30 AM - 9:45AM. *Medicine and Science in Sports and Exercise: Volume 37(5) Supplement May 2005 p. S284,* Copyright 2005 American College of Sports Medicine

40. Heather Hedrick Fink, Lisa A. Burgoon, Alan E. Mikesky. Practical Application in Sports Nutrition. Copyright 2006 by Jones and Bartlett Publishers, Inc.

41. Fatouros, Ioannis; Chatzinikolaou, Athanawsios; Jamurtas, Athanasios; Kallistratos; Illias; Baltzi, Maria; Douroudos, Ioannis; Fotinakis, Panagiotis; Taxildaris, Kiriakos; Vezyraki, Patra; Evangelou, Aggelos. The Effects of Self-Selected Music On Physiological Responses And performance During Cardiovascular Exercise: 555 Board #146 3:30 PM - 5:00 PM *Medicine and Science in Sports and Exercise: Volume 37(5) Supplement May 2005 p. S106,* Copyright 2006 American College of Sports Medicine

42. Flutem, Justin; Zukley, Linda; Lowndess, Joshua; Peel, Jeffrey, B.; Greenstone, Clinton L.; Angelopoulus, Gibbons, L. W.; Earnest, C. P.; Church T. S. Heart Rate Recovery After Maximal Exercise and Fitness Level Influences Cardiovascular Disease (CVD) and All-Cause Mortality Risk in Diabetic Men. *Medicine and Science in Sports and Exercise: Volume 34(5) Supplement 1 May 2002 p. S270,* Copyright 2006 American College of Sports Medicine

43. Qi Fu and Benjamin D. Levine. Cardiovascular Response to Exercise in Women. *Medicine and Science in Sports and Exercise 2005,* Copyright 2006 American College of Sports Medicine

44. Linn Goldberg, Diane L. Elliot and Kerry S. Kuehl. Cardiovascular Changes at Rest and During Mixed Static and Dynamic Exercise after Weight Training. *Journal of Applied Sport Science research* 2(3) pp. 42-43, 1998

45. Linn Goldberg, Diane L. Elliot and Kerry S. Kuehl. A Comparison of the Cardiovascular Effects of Running and Weight Training. *J. Strength Cond. Res. 8(4), 219-224, 2002.* Copyright 2002 National Strength and Conditioning Association.

46. Lincoln A. Gotshalk, Richard A. Berger, and William J. Kraemer. Cardiovascular Responses to a High Volume Continuous Circuit Resistance Training Protocol. *Medicine and Science in Sports and Exercise: Volume 18(4) p. 760-764, 2004,* Copyright 2006 American College of Sports Medicine

47. Guerra, S. C.; Ribiero, J. C.; Teixeira-Pinto, A; Duarte, J. A.; Mota, J. A. Relation Between Obesity and Cardiovascular Risk Factors in Portuguese Children. *Medicine and Science in Sports and Exercise: Volume 34(5) Supplement May 2002 p. S283,* Copyright 2005 American College of Sports Medicine

48. Gutlin, B.; Kang, H -S.; Howe, C.; Litaker, M.; Allison, J.; Hoffman, W.; Le, N -A.; Barbeau, P. Relation of Fasting Insulin with Cardiovascular Fitness, Total Body Fatness and Visceral Adipose Tissue in 8-11 Year Old Black Girls. *Medicine and Science in Sports and Exercise: Volume 34(5) Supplement 1 May 2002 p. S51,* Copyright 2006 American College of Sports Medicine

49. Hamilton, Janet; Lauer, Cynthia; Poudevigne, Melanie. Cardiovascular Risk Profiles of Collegiate Undergraduate Students: 1989 Board #128 3:30 PM - 5:00 PM. *Medicine and*

Science in Sports and Exercise: Volume 37(5) Supplement May 2005 p. S384-S385, Copyright 2006 American College of Sports Medicine

50. Jorn Wulff Helge. Long-Term fat diet adaptation effects on performance, training capacity, and fat utilization. *Medicine and Science in Sports and Exercise: Volume 34(9) p. 1499-1504,* Copyright 2002 American College of Sports Medicine

51. Hollander, D.B.; Ciano-Federoff, L; Perma, F. M.; Larkin, K. T. Social Support Buffers Cardiovascular and Perceptual Responses to Exercise and Recovery But Not Anticipation to Exercise. *Medicine and Science in Sports and Exercise: Volume 33(5) Supplement 1 May 2005 p. S261,* Copyright 2006 American College of Sports Medicine

52. Edward T. Howley, B. Don Franks. Health Fitness Instructors Handbook - 3rd Edition. Human Kinetics, Copyright 1997, 1992, 1986 by Edward T. Howley and B. Don Franks

53. Gang Hu, Heikki Pekkarinen, Osmo Hanninen, Zhijie Yu, Zeyu Guo, and Hiuguang Tian. Commuting, Leisure-time Physical Activity, and Cardiovascular Risk Factors in China. *Medicine and Science in Sports and Exercise: Volume 34(2) p. 234-238, 2002* Copyright 2006 American College of Sports Medicine

54. Rommie J. Hughes, Glen O. Johnson, Terry J. Housh, Joe P. Weir, and James E. Kinder. The Effect of Submaximal Treadmill Running on Serum Testosterone Levels. *J. Strength Cond. Res. 10(4), 224-227, 1996.* Copyright 1996 National Strength and Conditioning Association

55. Hui, S. C.; Thomas, G. N.; Tomlinson, B. Physical Activity, Fitness and Cardiovascular Risk Factors in Middle-Age Chinese Women. *Medicine and Science in Sports and Exercise: Volume*

34(5) Supplement 1 May 2002 p. S122, Copyright 2006 American College of Sports Medicine

56. Humphries, M. C.; Barbeau, P.; Litaker, M. S.; Gutlin, B. Cardiovascular Fitness(CVF) in Black and White Teens: Relations to Physical Activity (PA), and Sedentariness (SED). *Medicine and Science in Sports and Exercise: Volume 35(5) Supplement 1 May 2003 p. S180,* Copyright 2006 American College of Sports Medicine

57. Ihmels, Michelle; Eisenmann, Joey C.; Welk, Gregory J. Aerobic Fitness, Fatness and Cardiovascular Disease Risk Factors Among Australian Youth: 1504 9:45 AM - 10:00 AM. *Medicine and Science in Sports and Exercise: Volume 37(5) Supplement May 2005 p. S285,* Copyright 20056American College of Sports Medicine

58. Ishikawa-Takata, Kazuko: Ohta, Toshiki; Tanaka, Hirofumi. Physical Activity and Development of Hypertension and Diabetes: Dose-Response Relations. *Medicine and Science in Sports and Exercise: Volume 36(5) Supplement May 2004 p. S85 ,* Copyright 2006 American College of Sports Medicine

59. Mikel Izquierdo, Keijo Hakkinen, Javier Ibanez, Alanze Anton, Miriam Garrues, Maite Ruesta, and Exteban M. Gorostiaga. Effects of Strength Training on Submaximal and Maximal Endurance Performance Capacity in Middle-Aged and Older Men. *J. Strength Cond. Res. 17(1), 129-139, 2003.* Copyright 2003 National Strength and Conditioning Association

60. Izquierdo, Mikel; Ibanes, Javier; Hakkinen, Keifo, Kraemer, William J.; Larrion, Jose L.; Gorostiaga, Esteban M. Ounce Weekly Combined Resistance and Cardiovascular Training in Healthy Older Men. *Medicine and Science in Sports and Exercise: Volume 36(3) p. 435-443, 2004 ,* Copyright 2006 American College of Sports Medicine

61. Izquierdo, M.; Ibanes, J.; Hakkinen, K.; Kraemer, W.; Gorostiaga, E. M. Specificity of Long-Term Neuromuscular and Cardiovascular Adaptations. *Medicine and Science in Sports and Exercise 35(5) Supplement 1 May 2003 p. S291*, Copyright 2006 American College of Sports Medicine

62. Jackson, V.J.; Glass, S. C.. Influence of Fitness Level on the Relative Intensity for Peak Fat Utilization 85. *Medicine and Science in Sports and Exercise: Volume 23(5) Supplement 1 May 2001 p. S254*, Copyright 2006 American College of Sports Medicine

63. Jacobson, B. H. Relationship between Aerobic Exercise Frequency and Annual Health Related Absenteeism. *Medicine and Science in Sports and Exercise: Volume 36(5) Supplement May 2004 p. S135*, Copyright 2006 American College of Sports Medicine

64. Janssen, Ian; Katzmarzyk, Peter T.; Church Timothy S.; Blair Steven N. Predicting Cardiovascular Disease Mortality in Men Using Cardiorespiratory Fitness and Other Risk Factor Categories. *Medicine and Science in Sports and Exercise: Volume 36(5) Supplement May 2004 p. S135*, Copyright 2006 American College of Sports Medicine

65. Ronald E. Johnston, Timothy J. Quinn, Robert Kertzer, and Neil B. Vroman. Strength Training in Female Distance Runners: Impact on Running Economy. *J. Strength Cond. Res. 11(4), 224-229, 1998.* Copyright 1998 National Strength and Conditioning Association

66. Kang, Jie; Foffman, Jay; Tatamess, Nicholas; Faigenbaum, Avery; Falvo, Michael. Gender Differences in Fat Utilization: Effect of Exercise Intensity: 1418 4:30 PM - 4:45 PM *Medicine and Science in Sports and Exercise: Volume 37(5) Supplement May 2005 p. S275*, Copyright 2006 American College of Sports Medicine

67. Ketelhut, K.S.; Bittman, F.; Ketelhut, R.G. Fitness, Fatness and Cardiovascular Risk Profile - A Retrospective Study Among 11-13 Year Old Students in Germany. *Medicine and Science in Sports and Exercise: Volume 34(5) Supplement 1 May 2002 p. S227*, Copyright 2006 American College of Sports Medicine

68. Kilpatrick, M ; Bartholomew, J ; Hebert, E. Behavioral Regulations in Physical Activity: A Comparison of Sport and Exercise Motivation, *Medicine & Science in Sports & Exercise 35(5) Supplement 1 May 2003 p. S150*, Copyright 2006 American College of Sports Medicine

69. Kingsley, James D.; Panton, Lynn B.; Toole, Tonya; Moffat, Robert; Kushnick, Michael; Haymes, Emily. Cardiovascular Risk Factors of Low Socioeconomic Overweight and Obese Women Following 12-Month Use of Pedometers: 1510 9:45Am - 10:00 AM. *Medicine and Science in Sports and Exercise: Volume 37(5) Supplement May 2005 p. S286,* Copyright 2006 American College of Sports Medicine

70. Harold W. Kohl III. Physical Activity and Cardiovascular disease: Evidence for a dose response. *Medicine and Science in Sports and Exercise: Volume 33(6) Supplement May 2001 p. S472-S483,* Copyright 2006 American College of Sports Medicine

71. Komatsu, N.; Iwane, H.; Shimomitsu, T.; Katsumura, T.; Ohya, Y.; Homaoka, T.; Odagiri, Y.; Fujimami J. A Recommended Exercise Time and Frequency to Reduce Coronary Risk Factors in Japanese Males 82. *Medicine and Science in Sports and Exercise: Volume 28(5) Supplement May 1996 p. 14,* Copyright 2006 American College of Sports Medicine

72. Len Kravitz, Larry Greene, Zachary Burkett, and Jataporn Wongsathikun. Cardiovascular Response to Punching Tempo. *Strength Cond. Res.* 17(1), 104-108, Copyright 2003 National Strength and Conditioning Association

73. Heikki Kyrolainen, Paavo V. Komi, and Alain Belli. Changes in Muscle Activity Patterns and Kinetics With Increasing Running Speed. *J. Strength Cond. Res. 13(4), 400-406, 1999.* Copyright 1999 National Strength and Conditioning Association

74. I-min Lee and Patrick J. Skerrett. Physical Activity and All-Cause Mortality: What is the Dose-Response Relation? *Medicine and Science in Sports and Exercise: Volume 33(6) Suppl. 2001 p. S459-471,* Copyright 2006 American College of Sports Medicine

75. Leninrad, L. I.; Salmon, R.D.; English, C. D.; Faircloth, G.C.; Mitchell, B. S.; Saxon, W. E.; Reid, K. S.; Franklin, B. A., Franklin, N. F. Clinical Effectiveness of a Community-Based Cardiovascular Risk Reeducation Program in Participants With and Without Arthritis. *Medicine and Science in Sports and Exercise: Volume 34(5) Supplement 1 May 2002 p. S159,* Copyright 2006 American College of Sports Medicine

76. Liang, Michael T.; Moreno, Alejandro M.; Young Lisa K.; Chaung, William. Effects of Panaz Notoginseng on Aerobic Endurance and Cardiovascular Parameters in Adult Humans: 220 Board #127 9:30AM - 11:00AM. *Medicine and Science in Sports and Exercise: Volume 37(5) Supplement May 2005 p. S41,* Copyright 2006 American College of Sports Medicine

77. Lovell, Richard J.; Pout, Martin J.; Ryder, James J. Beverage Temperature: Effects upon Cardiovascular and Thermoregulatory Responses to Endurance Activity. *Medicine and Science in Sports and Exercise: Volume 36(5) Supplement May 2004 p. S315,* Copyright 2006 American College of Sports Medicine

78. Lowndess, Joshua; Zukley, Linda; Melton, Renee; FlutemJustin; Greenstone, Clinton L.; Anegelopoulos, Theodore J.; Rippe, JamesM. C-reactive Protein Has A Greater Association With Novel Cardiovascular Disease Risk Factors Than Components of The Metabolic Syndrome: 1993 Board #132 3:30 PM - 5:00 PM.

Medicine and Science in Sports and Exercise: Volume 37(5) Supplement May 2005 p. S385, Copyright 2006 American College of Sports Medicine

79. MacTaggart, J. N., Hansen, M. R.; Kolhorst, F. W. Effect of the Access Fat Conversion Activity Bar on Fat Utilization and Time to Exhaustion 292. *Medicine and Science in Sports and Exercise: Volume 29(5) Supplement 1 May 1997 p. S342,* Copyright 2006 American College of Sports Medicine

80. Malloy-McFall, J: Dochstander, L; Otterstetter, R; Lowery, L; Ziegenfuss, T; Caine, N; Glickman, E.L. Effect ofan Herbal Supplement on Thermoregulatory, Cardiovascular, and Metabolic Responses During Submaximal Exerciese. *Medicine and Science in Sports and Exercise: Volume 34(5) Supplement 1 May 2002 p. S225,* Copyright 2006 American College of Sports Medicine

81. Mummery, W.K.: Capperchione, C. M.;Schofeld, G. M. Dose-Response Effects of Physical Activity on Mental Health Status in Older Adults. *Medicine and Science in Sports and Exercise: Volume 35(5) Supplement 1 May 2003 p. S215,* Copyright 2006 American College of Sports Medicine

82. Matteson, E.; Carlson, B.; Kenyon, A.; Westbrook; Gagnet, A.; Vito, J.; Fluery, J. Frequency and Intensity of Self Reported Physical Activity Among Older Adults With Diagnosed Coronary Heart Disease. *Medicine and Science in Sports and Exercise: Volume 33(5) Supplement 1 May 2001 p. S62,* Copyright 2006 American College of Sports Medicine

83. Martin, D.; Perri, M.; Limacher, M.; Duncan, G.; Ketterson, T.; Syderman, S.; Anton, S.; Yang, M. Dose Response of Exercise Intensity and Frequency on Fitness and CAD Risk Factors. *Medicine and Science in Sports and Exercise: Volume 34(5)*

Supplement 1 May 2002 p. S69, Copyright 2006 American College of Sports Medicine

84. Mays, W.A.; Lockwood S.K.; Dopser, S. J.; Knilans, T.K.; Kirk, S; Daniels S.R.; Claytor, R. P., Obese Children Exhibit Similar Improvements in Submaximal Cardiovascular Function with and Without Improvements inVO2 Max. *Medicine and Science in Sports and Exercise: Volume 33(5) Supplement May 2001 p. S109,* Copyright 2006 American College of Sports Medicine

85. William D. McArdle, Frank I. Katch, Victor L. Katch. Exercise Physiology, Energy, Nutrition, and Human performance, 4th Edition. Pgs. 508-509, 652, Copyright 1996, Williams & Wilkins,

86. Mensink, Gert B. M.: Heerstrass, Desiree W.; Neppelenbroek, Sabine E.; Schuit, Albertine J.; Bellach, Barbel-Maria. Intensity, Duration, and Frequency of Physical Activity and Coronary Risk Factors. *Medicine and Science in Sports and Exercise: Volume 29(9) September 1997 pp. S1192-1198,* Copyright 2006 American College of Sports Medicine

87. Mesa J. L. M.; Ruiz, J. R.; Gutierzz, A; Gonzales-Grossc, M.; Moreno, L. A.; Perez-Prieto, R.; Hernandez, J. J. Does the Present Aerobic Fitness in Adolescents Guarantee Cardiovascular Health? *Medicine and Science in Sports and Exercise: Volume 35(5) Supplement 1 May 2003 p. S179,* Copyright 2006 American College of Sports Medicine

88. Thomas J. Michaud, David K. Brennan, Robert P. Wilder, and Nestor W. Sherman. Aquarunning and Gains Cardiorespiratory Fitness. *J. Strength Cond. Res.* 9(2), 78-74, 1995. Copyright 2006 National Strength and Conditioning Association

89. Mindy Millard-Stafford, Phillip B. Sparling, Linda B. Rosskopf, and Linda J. DiCarlo. Differences in Peak Physiological Responses During Running, Cycling and Swimming. *Journal of Applied*

Sport Science and Research. 5(4), 213-218 1991, Copyright 2002 National Strength and Conditioning Association

90. Marie Murphy, Alan Nevill, Charlotte Neville, Stuart Biddle, and Adrianne Hardman. Accumulating Brisk Walking for Fitness, Cardiovascular Risk, and Psychological Health. *Medicine and Science in Sports and Exercise: Volume 34(9) Supplement May 2004 p. 1468-1474,* Copyright 2006 American College of Sports Medicine

91. Murtagh, E. M.; Boreham, C.A. G.; Sprevak, D.; Murphy, M. H. Effects of 60-Min Brisk Walking Per Week on Cardiovascular Risk. *Medicine and Science in Sports and Exercise: Volume 35(5) Supplement 1 May 2003 p. S71,* Copyright 2006 American College of Sports Medicine

92. Naylor, Louisse; Amolda, Leonard; Playford,David; Deague, Jenny; O'Driscoll, Gerry, Fitzsimons, Martin; Green, Danny. Effects of Exercise Training on Cardiovascular Function and Structure in Elite Athletes. *Medicine and Science in Sports and Exercise: Volume 36(5) Supplement May 2004 p. S330-S331,* Copyright 2006 American College of Sports Medicine

93. Pekka Oja. Dose Response Between Total Volume of Physical Activity and Health and Fitness. *Medicine and Science in Sports and Exercise: Volume 33(6) Suppl., 2001 p. S428-437,* Copyright 2006 American College of Sports Medicine

94. Okazaki, Kazunobu; Iwasaki, Ken-Ichi; Palmer, Dean; Martini, Emily; Witkowski, Sarah; Prased, Anand; Arbeb- Zadeh, Armin; Fu, Qi; Zhang, Rong; Levine Benjamin D. Effects of Identical Training Volume and Intensity on Cardiovascular Variability in Young and Older Subjects. *Medicine and Science in Sports and Exercise: Volume 36(5) Supplement May 2004 p. S86,* Copyright 2006 American College of Sports Medicine

95. Okazaki, Kazunobu; Prased, Anand; Palmer, M. Dean; Martini, Emily R.; Arbab-Zadeh, Armin; Fu, Qi; Iwasaki, Ken-ichi; Zhang, Rong; Levine, Benjamin D. Dose Response of The Cardiovascular Adaptations to Endurance Training in Healthy Seniors:2175 9:30 AM - 9:45 AM. *Medicine and Science in Sports and Exercise: Volume 37(5) Supplement May 2005 p. S417*, Copyright 2006 American College of Sports Medicine

96. Stephen K. Oliver, and Mark S. Tremblay. Effects of a Sports Nutrition Bar on Endurance Running Performance. *J. Strength Cond. Res.* 16(1), 152-156, Copyright 2002 National Strength and Conditioning Association

97. Orri, Julia C.; Carter, Steven-Ryder; Brown Crystal D.; White Lesley J. C-reactive Protein, Fitness, and Cardiovascular Risk in College Students: 399 Board #8. *Medicine and Science in Sports and Exercise: Volume 37(5) Supplement May 2005 p. S70,* Copyright 2006 American College of Sports Medicine

98. Renza Perini, Nadine Fisher, Arsenio Veisteinas, and David R. Pendergast. Aerobic Training and Cardiovascular Responses at Rest and During Exercise in Older Men and Women. *Medicine and Science in Sports and Exercise: Volume 34(4) p. 700-708, 2005 ,* Copyright 2006 American College of Sports Medicine

99. Pritzlaff, C.j.; Widerman, L.; Weltman, J.Y.; Gaesser, G/A/; Hartman, M.L. ; Veldhuis, J.d. ; Weltman A. The Lactate Threshold and Carbohydrate and Fat Utilization During Exercise: Evaluation of the Crossover Concept. *Medicine and Science in Sports and Exercise: Volume 29(5) Supplement 1 May 1997 p. S342,* Copyright 2006 American College of Sports Medicine

100. Ramadan, J. M.; Barac-Nieto, M. Effects of Frequency of Physical Activity on Body Composition and Fitness in Adult Females. *Medicine and Science in Sports and Exercise: Volume 33(5)*

Supplement 1 May 2001 p. S74, Copyright 2006 American College of Sports Medicine

101. Ramadan, J. M.; Barac-Nieto, M. Effects of Reported Frequency of Physical Activity on Aerobic Fitness and Body Composition in Males and Females. *Medicine and Science in Sports and Exercise: Volume 34(5) Supplement 1 May 2002 p. S295,* Copyright 2006 American College of Sports Medicine

102. Resaland, G. K.; Aasen, S. B.; Hallen, J. External Nasal Strips Do Not Alter Cardio-Respiratory Response During Submaximal and Maximal Exercise. *Medicine and Science in Sports and Exercise: Volume 33(5) Supplement 1 May, 2001 p. S60,* Copyright 2006 American College of Sports Medicine

103. Caroline R. Richardson, Andrea M. Kriska, Paula M. Lantz, and Rodney A. Hayward. Physical Activity and Mortality across Cardiovascular Disease Risk Groups. *Medicine and Science in Sports and Exercise: Volume 36(11) p. 1923-1929, 2004 ,* Copyright 2006 American College of Sports Medicine

104. Richardson, Melanie T.; Ruiz, Roberto; Hughes, Cynthia L.; Sipos, Maurice L.; Williams, Thomas J. Self-Reported Exercise Frequency Predicts the Accuracy of Using a Circumference Test in Senior Military Leaders. *Medicine and Science in Sports and Exercise: Volume 36(5) Supplement May 2004 p. S262,* Copyright 2006 American College of Sports Medicine

105. Riebe, Deborah; Morrell, Candice A.; Ward, Christie L.; Blissmer, Bryan; Maher, Joseph F.: Silva Jessica E. The Effects of Exercise Order on the Perceptual Responses to Cardiovascular and Resistance Exercise. *Medicine and Science in Sports and Exercise: Volume 36(5) Supplement May 2004 p. S133,* Copyright 2006 American College of Sports Medicine

106. Theodore J. Rippe, James M. Association Between C-Reactive Protein and Cardiovascular Fitness in Obese Individuals: 1995 Board #134 3:30 PM - 5:00 PM. *Medicine and Science in Sports and Exercise: Volume 37(5) Supplement May 2005 p. S386,* Copyright 2006 American College of Sports Medicine

107. Robert Ross and Ian Janssen. Physical Activity, Total and Regional Obesity: Dose-Response Considerations. *Medicine and Science in Sports and Exercise: Volume 33(6) Suppl., 2001 p. S521-S527,* Copyright 2006 American College of Sports Medicine

108. Rowland, Thomas W.; Pober, David; Garrison, Anne. Determinants of Cardiovascular Drift in Euhydrated Prepubertal Boys: 1146 Board #1. *Medicine and Science in Sports and Exercise: Volume 37(5) Supplement May 2005 p. S216,* Copyright 2006 American College of Sports Medicine

109. Alberto Ruiz and Nestor W. Sherman. An Evaluation of the Accuracy of the American College of Sports Medicine Metabolic Equation for Estimating the Oxygen Cost of Running. *Strength Cond. Res.* 13(3), 219-223, Copyright 1999 National Strength and Conditioning Association

110. Savonen, K.; Lakka, T. A.; Laukkanen, J.; Salonen, J. T.; Rauramaa, R. Submaximal Oxygen Pulse Predicts Total and Cardiovascular Mortality in Men. *Medicine and Science in Sports and Exercise: Volume 34(5) Supplement 1 May 2002 p. S123,* Copyright 2006 American College of Sports Medicine

111. Saunders, M. J.; Flohr, J. A.; Todd, M. K.. A Comparison of the Benefits of Cardioresistance Training Versus Cardiovascular and Resistance Training. *Medicine and Science in Sports and Exercise: Volume 34(5) Supplement 1 May 2002 p. S26,* Copyright 2006 American College of Sports Medicine

112. Timothy C. Schell, Glen Wright, Paul Martino, Jeff Ryder, and Bruce W. Craig. Postexercise Glucose, Insulin, and C-Peptide Responses to Carbohydrate Supplementation: Running vs. Resistance Exercise. *J. Strength Cond. Res.* 13(4), 372-380, Copyright 1999 National Strength and Conditioning Association

113. Schoefield, L.; Mummery, W.K. Descriptive Study of Pedometer-Determined Ambulatory Activity and Selected Cardiovascular Disease Risk Factors in Adolescent Girls. *Medicine and Science in Sports and Exercise: Volume 35(5) Supplement 1 May 2003 p. S341,* Copyright 2006 American College of Sports Medicine

114. Roy J. Shephard. Absolute Versus Relative Intensity of Physical Activity in a Dose-Response Context. *Medicine and Science in Sports and Exercise: Volume 33(6) Suppl., 2001 pp. S400-418,* Copyright 2006 American College of Sports Medicine

115. Nestor W. Sherman. Development of a Generalized Model to Estimate the Energy Cost of Walking and Running for Healthy Adults. *Strength Cond. Res.* 12(1), 33-36, Copyright 1998 National Strength and Conditioning Association

116. Sinclair, D. R.;; Essig, F.; Swank, A. M.; Durham, M. P.; Adams. K.J.; Kipp, R.L. Cardiovascular Risk Factors for University Faculty and Staff: Comparative Analysis. *Medicine and Science in Sports and Exercise: Volume 33(5) Supplement 1 May 2001 p. S155,* Copyright 2006 American College of Sports Medicine

117. Parco M. Siu, Stephen H.S Wong, John G. Morris, Ching W. Lam, Pak K Chung, and Susan Chung. Effect of Frequency of Carbohydrate Feedings on Recovery and Subsequent Endurance Run. *Medicine and Science in Sports and Exercise: Volume 36(2) p. 315-323,* Copyright 2004 American College of Sports Medicine

118. Spalding, Thomas W.; Lyon Lewis A., Hatfield, Bradley D. Relative Efficacy of Aerobic Training and Stress Management in Lowering

Cardiovascular Activity During Psychological Stress. *Medicine and Science in Sports and Exercise: Volume 36(5) Supplement May 2004 p. S90,* Copyright 2006 American College of Sports

119. Barry A. Spiering, Meredith H. Wilson, Daniel A. Judelson, and Kenneth W. Rundell. Evaluation of Cardiovascular Demands of Game Play and Practice in Women's Ice Hockey. . *Strength Cond. Res.* 17(2), 329-333, 2003. Copyright 2003 National Strength and Conditioning Association

120. Waneen W. Spirduso and D. Leilani Cronin. Exercise Dose-Response Effects on Quality of Life and Independent Living in Older Adults. *Medicine and Science in Sports and Exercise: Volume 33(6) Suppl., 2001 p. S598-S608,* Copyright 2006 American College of Sports Medicine

121. Robert Stanton, Peter R. Reaburn, and Brendan Humphries. The Effect of Short-Term Swiss Ball Training on Core Stability and Running Economy. *J. Strength Cond. Res. 18(3), 522-528, 2004.* Copyright 2004 National Strength and Conditioning Association

122. Stephenson, Claire E.; George, Keith P.; Cable Nigel T. Cardiovascular Responses to a 6-Month Aerobic Training Programme in Post-menopausal Females: 1155 Board #10 3:30 PM - 5:00 PM. *Medicine and Science in Sports and Exercise: Volume 37(5) Supplement May 2005 p. S218,* Copyright 2006 American College of Sports Medicine

123. Michael H. Stone, William A. Sands, Jon Carlock, Sam Callan, Des Dickie, Karen Daigle, John Cotton, Sarah L. Smith, and Michael Hartman. The Importance of Isometric Maximum Strength and Peak Rate-of-Force Development in Sprint Cycling. *J. Strength Cond. Res. 18(4), 878-884, 2004.* Copyright 2004 National Strength and Conditioning Association

124. David Q. Thomas, Beth M. Larson, Michele R. Rahija, and Steven T. McCaw. Nasal Strips Do Not Affect Cardiorespiratory Measures During Recovery From Anaerobic Exercise. *J. Strength Cond. Res. 15(3), 341-343, 2001.* Copyright 2001 National Strength and Conditioning Association

125. Inger Thune and Anne-Sofie Furberg. Physical Activity and Cancer Risk: Dose-Response and Cancer, All Sites and Site Specific. *Medicine and Science in Sports and Exercise: Volume 33(6) Supplement May 2001 p. S530-S550,* Copyright 2006 American College of Sports Medicine

126. Todd, M. K.; Flohr, J. A.; Saunders, M. J. Comparison of Cardioresistance, Resistance and Cardiovascular Training on Selected Health Indices. *Medicine and Science in Sports and Exercise: Volume 34(5) Supplement 1 May 2002 p. S23,* Copyright 2006 American College of Sports Medicine

127. Nebojsa Nash Toskovic, Daniel Blessing, and Henry N. Williford. The Effect of Experience and Gender on Cardiovascular and Metabolic Responses With Dynamic Tae Kwon Do Exercise. *J. Strength Cond. Res. 16(2), 278-285, 2002.* Copyright 2002 National Strength and Conditioning Association

128. Amanda M. Turner, Matt Owings, and James A Schwane. Improvements in Running Economy After 6 Weeks of Plyometric Training. *J. Strength Cond. Res. 17(1), 60-67, 2003.* Copyright 2003 National Strength and Conditioning Association

129. Twisk, J. W. R.; Mechelen, W.; Kemper, H.C.G. Physical Activity and Physical Fitness During Adolescence and Cardiovascular Risk Factors at Adult Age. *Medicine and Science in Sports and Exercise: Volume 34(5) Supplement 1 May 2002 p. S254,* Copyright 2006 American College of Sports Medicine

130. Umstattd, Michelle Renee; McIver, Kerry L.; Smith, Sharon; Dubose, Katrina D.; Ainsworth, Barbara E. Cardiovascular Disease Risk Factors and Physical Activity Status Among Older Adults, 2001 BRFSS. *Medicine and Science in Sports and Exercise: Volume 36(5) Supplement May 2004 p. S192-S193,* Copyright 2006 American College of Sports Medicine

131. Ilkka M. Vuori. Dose-Response of Physical Activity and Low Back Pain, Osteoarthritis, and Osteoporosis. *Medicine and Science in Sports and Exercise: Volume 33(6) Supplement May 2001 p. S551-S586,* Copyright 2006 American College of Sports Medicine

132. Whitt, M.; Ainsworth, B.; Stolarzcyk, L.; Levin S.; Irwin, M.; Hootman, J.; Orri, J.; Heyward, V. Frequency of Moderate Activity in Minority Women. *Medicine and Science in Sports and Exercise: Volume 35(5) Supplement 1 May 2003 p. S179,* Copyright 2006 American College of Sports Medicine

133. Wickel, Eric E.; Eisenmann, Joey C.; Welk, Gregory J. Adolescent Aerobic Fitness and Adult Cardiovascular Disease Risk Factors: The Aerobics Center Longitudinal Study. *Medicine and Science in Sports and Exercise: Volume 30(5) Supplement May 1998 p. 218,* Copyright 2006 American College of Sports Medicine

134. Jack H. Wilmore. Dose-Response: Variation With Age, Sex, and Health Status. *Medicine and Science in Sports and Exercise: Volume 33(6) Suppl., 2001 p. S622-S634,* Copyright 2006 American College of Sports Medicine

135. Wingo, Jonathan; Lafrenze, Andrew; Stueck, Matt, Cureton, Kirk. Effects of Cardiovascular Drift on Maximal Oxygen Uptake: Influence of Hydration. *Medicine and Science in Sports and Exercise: Volume 36(5) Supplement May 2004 p. S331,* Copyright 2006 American College of Sports Medicine

136. Jonathan E. Wingo, Andrew J. Lafrenz, Mathew S. Gango, Gaylen L. Edwards, and Kirk J. Cureton. Cardiovascular Drift Is Related to Reduced Maximal Oxygen Uptake during Heat Stress. *Medicine and Science in Sports and Exercise: Volume 37(2) p. 248-255. 2005,* Copyright 2006 American College of Sports Medicine

137. Wingo, Jonathan; Lafrenze, Andrew; Stueck, Matt, Cureton, Kirk. Effects of Cardiovascular Drift on Maximal Oxygen Uptake at Two Ambient Tempetures:893 Board #115 9:00 AM - 10:30 AM. *Medicine and Science in Sports and Exercise: Volume 37(5) Supplement May 2005 p. S169,* Copyright 2006 American College of Sports Medicine

138. Robert H. Wood, Rafael Reyes, Michael A. Welcsh, Jennifer Favaloro-Sabatier, Manning Sabatier, C. Matthew Lee, Lisa G. Johnson, and Pleasant F. Hooper. Concurrent Cardiovascular and Resistance Training in Healthy Older Adults. *Medicine and Science in Sports and Exercise: Volume 33(10) p. 1751-1758, 2001 ,* Copyright 2006 American College of Sports Medicine

139. Matthew A. Wyon and Emma Redding. Physiological Monitoring of Cardiorespiratory Adaptations During Rehearsal and Performance of Contemporary Dance. *J. Strength Cond. Res.* 19(4), 611-614, 2005. Copyright 2005 National Strength and Conditioning Association

140. Annesi JJ. *Goal-Setting Protocol in Adherence to Exercise by Italian Adults.* Percept Mot Skills. 2002 Apr;94(2):453-8. / PMID 12027338 [PubMed - indexed for MEDLINE]

141. Bess H. Marcus, PhD & Beth A. Lewis, PhD. *Physical Activity and The Stages of Motivational Readiness for Change Model.* Presidents Counsel of Physical Fitness and Sports,

Research Digest, Series 4, No. 1, March 2003

142. Kilpatrick, M ; Bartholomew, J ; Hebert, E. *Behavioral Regulations in Physical Activity: A Comparison of Sport and Exercise Motivation*, Medicine & Science in Sports & Exercise May 2003, 35:5 Supplement 1 p S150 /Copyright American College of Sports Medicine 2004

143. Ben C. Sporer and Howard A. Wenger. Effects of Aerobic Exercise on Strength Performance Following Various Periods of Recover. *J. Strength Cond. Res. 17(4),638-644, 2003.*

Bibliography: Section 3: Chapter 8

1.   Adams, K. J.; Snow, C. M.; Sevene, P. G.; Debeliso, M.; O'Shea, J. P.. Weightlifters Exhibit Greater Muscle Power and Lower Back Flexibility than Non-Weightlifters 1142. *Medicine and Science in Sports and Exercise: Volume 28(5) Supplement May 1996 p. 192*, Copyright 2005 American College of Sports Medicine

2.   Ahtikoski, A. M.; Koskinen, S.O.A.; Kovanen, V.; Virtanen, P.; Takala, T. E. S.. Regulation of Synthesis of Type I Collagen in Skeletal Muscle After Immobilization: Effect of Stretch 650

3.   American College of Sports Medicine. ACSM's Guidelines for Exercise Testing and Prescription, Sixth Edition; Senior Editor Barry A. Franklin, Associate Editor Mitchell H. Whaley and Edward T. Howley; Authors Gary J. Dalady…. [et. al.] Copyright 2001 American College of Sports Medicine

4.   Astrab J.; Small, E.; Kerner, M. S.. Muscle Strength and Flexibility in Young Elite Swimmers. . *Medicine and Science in Sports and Exercise: Volume 33(5) Supplement 1 May 2001 p. S342*, Copyright 2005 American College of Sports Medicine

5.   Araujo, C.. Body Flexibility Profile and Clustering Among Male and Female Elite Athletes. *Medicine and Science in Sports and Exercise: Volume 31(5) Supplement May 1999 p. S115,* Copyright 2005 American College of Sports Medicine

6.   Aruajo, C.; Pereira, M.; Farinatti, P.. Body Flexibility Profile From Childhood to Seniority - Data From 1874 Male and Female Subjects. *Medicine and Science in Sports and Exercise: Volume 30(5) Supplement May 1998 p. 115,* Copyright 2005 American College of Sports Medicine

7.   Araujo, Claudio G.; Araujo, Denise S.. Does Flexibility Always Decrease With Aging? - An 18-year Follow-up in 10 Women: 1223 Board #78 3:30 PM - 5:00 PM. *Medicine and Science in Sports and Exercise: Volume 37(5) Supplement May 2005 p. S234,* Copyright 2005 American College of Sports Medicine

8.   Thomas R. Baechle, Roger W. Earle. Essentials of Strength Training and Conditioning - 2nd Edition. Copyright 2000, 1994 National Strength and Condition Association

9.   Baltaci, G.; Tunay, V. Bayrakci. Shoulder Isokinetic Strength at Diagonal Pattern and Flexibility in F Professional Handball, Basketball and Volleyball Players. *Medicine and Science in Sports and Exercise: Volume 33(5) Supplement 1 May 2001 p. S245,* Copyright 2005 American College of Sports Medicine

10.   David M. Bazett-Jones, Jason B. Winchester, and Jeffrey M. McBride. Effect of Potentiation and Stretching on Maximal Force, Rate of Force Development, and Range of Motion. *J. Strength Cond. Res. 19(2), 421-426,* Copyright 2005 National Strength & Conditioning Association

11.   Joshua C. Barlow, Brian W. Benjamin, Patrick J. Birt, and Christopher J. Hughes. Shoulder Strength and Range-Of-Motion

Characteristics in Bodybuilders. *J. Strength Cond. Res. 16(3), 367-372*, Copyright 2002 National Strength & Conditioning Association

12. Beaudoin, C. M.; Blum, J. Whatley. An Examination of Flexibility and Running Economy in Female Collegiate Track Athletes. . *Medicine and Science in Sports and Exercise: Volume 33(5) Supplement 1 May 2001 p. S23,* Copyright 2005 American College of Sports Medicine

13. Barry Beedle, Chris Jessee and Micahel H. Stone. Flexibility Characteristics Among Athletes Who Weight Train. *Journal of Applied Sport Science Research 5(3) p. 150-154, 1991,* Copyright National Strength and Conditioning Association

14. David G. Behm, Andrew Bambury, Farrell Cahill, and Kevin Power. Effect of Acute Static Stretching on Force, Balance, Reaction Time, and Movement Time. *Medicine and Science in Sports and Exercise: Volume 36(8) p. 1397-1402, 2004,* Copyright 2005 American College of Sports Medicine

15. Belyea, B. C.; Sigg J. A.. Effect of Deep Heat, Cold, Active Exercise, and Stretching on Hamstring Flexibility. *Medicine and Science in Sports and Exercise: Volume 35(5) Supplement 1 May 2003 p. S108,* Copyright 2005 American College of Sports Medicine

16. Bernhardt, M.: Banzer, W. Flexibility Tests: Do They Discriminate Between Subjects With and Without Low-Back Pain? *Medicine and Science in Sports and Exercise: Volume 30(5) Supplement May 1998 p. 224,* Copyright 2005 American College of Sports Medicine

17. Colleen A. Boyle, Stephen P. Sawyers, Barbara E. Jensen, Samuel, A. Headley, and Tina M. Manos. The Effects of Yoga Training and a Single Bout of Yoga on Delayed Onset Muscle Soreness in the Lower Extremity. *J. Strength Cond. Res. 18(4), 723-729,* Copyright 2004 National Strength & Conditioning Association

18. Brill, Yaron; Rodd, Donald. The Effects of Stretching on Lower Body Strength and Functional Power Performance: 260 Board #167 9:30 AM - 11:00 AM. *Medicine and Science in Sports and Exercise: Volume 37(5) Supplement May 2005 p. S50,* Copyright 2005 American College of Sports Medicine

19. Brown, D. A.; Miller, W. C.. Strength and Flexibility in Middle- to Older-Aged Women are Far Below ACSM Norms. *Medicine and Science in Sports and Exercise: Volume 29(5) Supplement May 1997 p. 102,* Copyright 2005 American College of Sports Medicine

20. Browner-Elhanan, K.J.; Small, Eric; Coupey, Susan; Lee Ryan. Lower Limb Flexibility and Muscle Strength in Osgood Schlatter Disease. *Medicine and Science in Sports and Exercise: Volume 31(5) Supplement 1 May 1999 p. S359,* Copyright 2005 American College of Sports Medicine

21. Bulbulian, R.; Burke, J.; Kovach, M.; Ploutz-Snyder, R.. The Effect of Heteronomous Muscle Stretching on Motorneuron Excitability. *Medicine and Science in Sports and Exercise: Volume 31(5) Supplement May 1998 p. S136,* Copyright 2005 American College of Sports Medicine

22. Darren G. Burke, Christopher J. Culligan, Laurence E. Holt, and Natalie C. MacKinnon. Equipment Designed to Simulate Proprioceptive Neuromuscular Facilitation Flexibility Training. *J. Strength Cond. Res. 14(2), 135-139,* Copyright 2000 National Strength & Conditioning Association

23. Byrd, T.; Corneau, M. J.; Brown, L. E.; Greenwood, L.; Graves M. M.. The Effects of Two Different Stretching Forces on Viscoelastic Properties of the Hamstring Muscle Group. *Medicine and Science in Sports and Exercise: Volume 34(5) Supplement 1 May 2002 p. S151,* Copyright 2005 American College of Sports Medicine

24. Carvalho, Ana Cristina Gouvea; de Paula, Karla Campos; de Azavedo, Tania Maria Cordeiro; de Nobrega, Antonio Claudio Lucas. Relationship between Muscular Strength and Flexibility in Healthy Adults of Both Genders. . *Medicine and Science in Sports and Exercise: Volume 35(5) Supplement 1 May 2003 p. S279,* Copyright 2005 American College of Sports Medicine

25. 25. Celebi, M.M.; Zergeroglu, M.A.; Ergen. E.. The Effects of the Warm Up and Stretching Exercises on the Proprioception. *Medicine and Science in Sports and Exercise: Volume 31(1) January 1999 p. 190,* Copyright 2005 American College of Sports Medicine

26. J. Brian Church, Matthew S. Wiggins, F. Michael Moode, and Randall Christ. Effect of Warm-Up and Flexibility Treatments on Vertical Jump Performance. *J. Strength Cond. Res. 15(3), 332-336,* Copyright 2001 National Strength & Conditioning Association

27. Daniel Cipriani, Bobbie Abel, and Dayna Pirrwitz. A Comparison of Two Stretching Protocols on Hip Range of Motion: Implications for Total Daily Stretch Duration. *J. Strength Cond. Res. 17(2), 274-278,* Copyright 2003 National Strength & Conditioning Association

28. Clark, D. G.; Kinzey, S. J. Stretching Does Not Change Average EMG Values Measured During Maximal Voluntary Contractions. *Medicine and Science in Sports and Exercise: Volume 30(5) Supplement May 1998 p. 252,* Copyright 2005 American College of Sports Medicine

29. Michael A. Clark, Rodney J. Corn. NASM OPT Optimum Performance Training for the Fitness Professional, 2nd Edition. Copyright 2001, National Academy of Sports Medicine.

30. Michael A. Clark. Integrated Flexibility Training. Copyright 2001 National Academy of Sports Medicine.

31. Coles, Michael G.; Jones Harvey, Valerie N.; Greer, Felecia A.; Gilbert Wade D.. Effect of Sports Massage on Range of Motion, Peak Torque, and Time to Peak Torque: 1351 Board #206 2:00 PM - 3:30 PM. *Medicine and Science in Sports and Exercise: Volume 37(5) Supplement May 2005 p. S264,* Copyright 2005 American College of Sports Medicine

32. William I. Cornelius and Karen K Hayes. A Comparison of Single vs. Repeated MVIC Maneuvers Used in PNF Flexibility Techniques for Improvements in ROM. *Journal of Applied Sport Science Research 1(4) p. 72-73, 1987,* Copyright 1987 National Strength and Conditioning Association.

33. William I. Cornelius and Mary R. Rauschuber. The Relationship Between Isometric Contraction Durations and Improvement in Acute Hip Joint Flexibility. *Journal of Applied Sport Science Research 1(3) p. 39-41, 1987,* Copyright 1987 National Strength and Conditioning Association.

34. Cornwell, A.; Nelson, A. G.. The Acute Effects of Passive Stretching on Active Musculotendinous Stiffness 1594. *Medicine and Science in Sports and Exercise: Volume 29(5) Supplement May 1997 p. 281,* Copyright 2005 American College of Sports Medicine

35. Cornwell, A.; Nelson, A. G.; Sidaway, B.. Acute Effects of Passive Stretching on the Neuromechanical Behavior of the Triceps Surae Muscle Complex. *Medicine and Science in Sports and Exercise: Volume 31(5) Supplement May 1999 p. S221,* Copyright 2005 American College of Sports Medicine

36. Craib, Mitchell W.; Mitchell Vicki A.; Fields, Karl B.; Cooper, Theresa R.; Hopewell, Regina; Morgan Don W.. The Association Between Flexibility and Running Economy in Sub-Elite male Distance Runners. *Medicine and Science in Sports and Exercise: Volume 28(6) June 1996 2003 p. 737-743,* Copyright 2005 American College of Sports Medicine

37. Joel T. Cramer, Terry J. Housh, Glen O. Johnson, Joshua M. Miller, Jared W. Coburn, and Travis W. Beck. Acute Effects of Static Stretching on Peak Torque in Women. *J. Strength Cond. Res. 18(2), 236-241,* Copyright 2004 National Strength & Conditioning Association

38. Cramer, J. T.; Housh, T. J.; Johnson, G. O.; Miller, J.M.; Coburn, J. W.. The Acute Effects of Static Stretching on Peak Torque and EMG of The Stretched and Unstretched (Contralateral) Vastus Lateralis Muscles. *Medicine and Science in Sports and Exercise: Volume 35(5) Supplement 1 May 2003 p. S382,* Copyright 2005 American College of Sports Medicine

39. D. Scott Davis, Paul E. Ashley, Kristi L. McCale, Jerry A. McQuain, and Jaime M. Wine. The Effectiveness of 3 Stretching Techniques on Hamstring Flexibility Using Consistent Stretching Parameters. *J. Strength Cond. Res. 19(1), 27-32,* Copyright 2005 National Strength & Conditioning Association

40. Durham, M.; Stanziano, D.; Sandler, D.; Van Bemden, A.;Signorile, J. F.. Differences in Flexibility of Frail Elderly Fallers Versus Non-Fallers and Walking Aid Users Versus Non-Users. *Medicine and Science in Sports and Exercise: Volume 34(5) Supplement 1 May 2002 p. S175,* Copyright 2005 American College of Sports Medicine

41. Encarmacion, M. G.; Meyers, M. C.; Bloom, J.; Ryan, N. D.; Wooten J. S.. Upper Body Strength and Joint Range of Motion of Collegiate Male Golfers. *Medicine and Science in Sports and Exercise: Volume 30(5) Supplement May 1998 p. 240,* Copyright 2005 American College of Sports Medicine

42. Todd S. Ellenbecker and E. Paul Roetert. Effects of a 4-Month Season on Glenohumeral Joint Rotational Strength and Range of Motion in Female Collegiate Tennis Players. *J. Strength Cond. Res.*

16(1), 92-96, Copyright 2002 National Strength & Conditioning Association

43. Todd S. Ellenbecker, E. Paul Roetert, David S. Bailie, George J. Davies, and Scott W. Brown. Glenohumeral Joint Total Rotation Range of Motion in Elite Tennis Players and Baseball Pitchers. *Medicine and Science in Sports and Exercise: Volume 334(12) p. 2052-2056, 2002* Copyright 2005 American College of Sports Medicine

44. Sharon A. Evans, Terry J. Housh, Glen O Johnson, Janis Beaird, Dona J. Housh, and Merrel Pepper. Age-Specific Differences in the Flexibility of High School Wrestlers. *J. Strength Cond. Res. 7(1), 39-42*, Copyright 1993 National Strength & Conditioning Association

45. Tammy K. Evetovich, Natalie J. Nauman, Donovan S. Conley, and Jay B. Todd. Effect of Static Stretching of the Biceps Brachii on Torque, Electromyography and Mechanomyography During Concentric Isokinetic Muscle Actions. *J. Strength Cond. Res. 17(3), 484-488*, Copyright 2003 National Strength & Conditioning Association

46. Ewing, C.; Bloom, J.; Meyers, M. C.; Encarmacion, M. G.; Ryan, N. D.; Wooten J. S.; Nair, P. M.. Upper Body Strength and Joint Range of Motion of Elite, Adolescent Tae Kwon Do Athletes. *Medicine and Science in Sports and Exercise: Volume 31(5) Supplement May 1999 p. S170*, Copyright 2005 American College of Sports Medicine

47. Faigenbaum, Avery D.; Bellucci, Mario; Bernieri, Angelo; Bekker, Bart; Hoorens, Karlyn. Acute Effects of Pre-event Static Stretching on Fitness Performance in Children. *Medicine and Science in Sports and Exercise: Volume 36(5) Supplement May 2004 p. S356*, Copyright 2005 American College of Sports Medicine

48. Feland, J. B.; Myer, J. W.; Merril, R. M.. PNF Vs Static Stretch: Acute Responses in Hamstring Flexibility of Senior Athletes. *Medicine and Science in Sports and Exercise: Volume 33(5) Supplement 1 May 2001 p. S10,* Copyright 2005 American College of Sports Medicine

49. Ferber, R. ; Ostering, L. R.; Gravelle, D. Range of Motion and EMG Response to Proprioceptive Neuromuscular Facilitation Stretch Techniques in Trained and Untrained Older Adults. *Medicine and Science in Sports and Exercise: Volume 30(5) Supplement May 1998 p. S213,* Copyright 2005 American College of Sports Medicine

50. Fern, A.; Lendel, K.; Sezniak, E.; Boura, J.; Franklin, B. A.. Stretching Before or After Aerobic Exercise? *Medicine and Science in Sports and Exercise: Volume 33(5) Supplement 1 May 2001 p. S76,* Copyright 2005 American College of Sports Medicine

51. Iain M. Fletcher and Bethan Jones. The Effect of Different Warm-UP Stretch Protocols on 20 Meter Sprint Performance in Trained Rugby Union Players. *J. Strength Cond. Res. 18(4), 885-888,* Copyright 2004 National Strength & Conditioning Association

52. Fry, A. C.; McLellan, E.; Weiss, L. W.; Rosato, F. D.. The Effects of Static Stretching on Power and Velocity During the Bench Press Exercise. *Medicine and Science in Sports and Exercise: Volume 35(5) Supplement 1 May 2003 p. S264,* Copyright 2005 American College of Sports Medicine

53. Fowles, J. R.; Sale, D. G.. Time Course of Strength Deficit After Maximal Passive Stretch in Humans. *Medicine and Science in Sports and Exercise: Volume 29(5) Supplement May 1997 p. 26,* Copyright 2005 American College of Sports Medicine

54. Fowles, J. R.; Sale, D. G.. Time Course of Stress Relaxation with Repetitive Stretching of Human Plantarflexors. *Medicine and*

Science in Sports and Exercise: Volume 30(5) Supplement May 1998 p. 253, Copyright 2005 American College of Sports Medicine

55. Dan Funk, Ann M. Swank, Kent J. Adams, and Dwayne Treolo. Efficacy of Moist Heat Pack Application Over Static Stretching on Hamstring Flexibility. *J. Strength Cond. Res. 15(1), 123-126,* Copyright 2001 National Strength & Conditioning Association

56. Daniel C. Funk, Ann M. Swank, Benjamin M. Mikla, Todd A. Fagan, and Brian K. Farr. Impact of Prior Exercise on Hamstring Flexibility: A Comparison of Proprioceptive Neuromuscular Facilitation and Static Stretching. *J. Strength Cond. Res. 17(3), 489-492,* Copyright 2003 National Strength & Conditioning Association

57. Gappmaier, E.; Blake, B.; Jesse, D.; Overly, D.. Changes in Muscle Length or Stretch Tolerance? Effects of a 12 Month Hamstring Stretching Program. *Medicine and Science in Sports and Exercise: Volume 34(5) Supplement 1 May 2002 p. S153,* Copyright 2005 American College of Sports Medicine

58. Garrison, T.T.; Kluess, H. A.; Welsch, M.A.; Wood R. H.. Influence of Acute Stretching on Lower Limb Blood Flow. *Medicine and Science in Sports and Exercise: Volume 33(5) Supplement 1 May 2001 p. S209,* Copyright 2005 American College of Sports Medicine

59. Gerlach, K. E.; Burton, H. W.; Dorn, J. M.; Leddy, J. J.; White, S. C.; Horvath, P.J.. Fatigue, Balance, Running Mechanics and Flexibility as Risk Factors For Injury Among Female Runners. *Medicine and Science in Sports and Exercise: Volume 35(5) Supplement 1 May 2003 p. S279,* Copyright 2005 American College of Sports Medicine

60. Guillory, I. K.; Nelson A. G.; Cornwell, A.; Kokkonen, J.. Inhibition of Maximal Torque Production by Acute Stretching is Velocity Specific. *Medicine and Science in Sports and Exercise: Volume 30(5)*

Supplement May 1998 p. 101, Copyright 2005 American College of Sports Medicine

61. Gulgin, Heather R.; Armstrong, Charles W.. Hip Range of Motion Asymmetry in Elite Female Golfers: 606 Board #198 2:00 PM - 3:30 PM. . *Medicine and Science in Sports and Exercise: Volume 37(5) Supplement May 2005 p. S118,* Copyright 2005 American College of Sports Medicine

62. Harvey, D. M.. Flexibility of Elite Athletes Using the Modified Thomas Test 1545. *Medicine and Science in Sports and Exercise: Volume 29(5) Supplement May 1997 p. 271,* Copyright 2005 American College of Sports Medicine

63. Hasegawa, K. T.; Hori, S.; Suite, J.; Dawson M. L.. Effects of Stretching on Vastus Medial is and Vastus Lateralis. *Medicine and Science in Sports and Exercise: Volume 33(5) Supplement 1 May 2001 p. S10,* Copyright 2005 American College of Sports Medicine

64. David M. Hooper, Helen Hill, Wendy I. Drechsler, and Matthew C. Morrissey. Range of Motion Specificity Resulting From Closed and Open Kinetic Chain Resistance Training After Anterior Cruciate Ligament Reconstruction. *J. Strength Cond. Res. 16(3), 409-415,* Copyright 2002 National Strength & Conditioning Association

65. Hong, Youlian. Comparison of Flexibility and Heart Rate Responses Between Tai Chi Practioners and Nonpractitioners. *Medicine and Science in Sports and Exercise: Volume 31(5) Supplement May 1999 p. S160,* Copyright 2005 American College of Sports Medicine

66. David R. Hopkins, Werner W. K. Hoeger. A Comparison of the Sit-and -Reach Test and the Modified Sit-and-Reach Test in the Measurements of Flexibility for Males. *Journal of Applied Sport*

Science Research 1992, Volume 6, Number 1 pp. 7-10, Copyright 1992 National Strength and Conditioning Association

67. Edward T. Howley, B. Don Franks. Health Fitness Instructors Handbook - 3rd Edition. Human Kinetics, Copyright 1997, 1992, 1986 by Edward T. Howley and B. Don Franks

68. Hughes, H. G.; Schwellnus, M. P. The Effect of Static Stretch Duration and Frequency on Hamstring Musculotendinous Flexibility. *Medicine and Science in Sports and Exercise: Volume 30(5) Supplement May 1998 p. 25,* Copyright 2005 American College of Sports Medicine

69. Keefer, D.J.; Bassett, D. R. Jr.; Howley, E. T.; Johnson, K. R.. Relationship Between Lower-Body Flexibility and Running Economy on Level and Downhill Grades 395. *Medicine and Science in Sports and Exercise: Volume 28(5) Supplement May 1996 p. 66,* Copyright 2005 American College of Sports Medicine

70. Klein, D. A.. Does Flexibility Training Improve Physical Function in Assisted-Living Older Adults? *Medicine and Science in Sports and Exercise: Volume 33(5) Supplement 1 May 2001 p. S344,* Copyright 2005 American College of Sports Medicine

71. Duane V. Knudson, Guillermo J. Noffal, Rafael E. Bahamonde, Jeff A. Bauer, and John R. Blackwell. Stretching Has No Effect on Tennis Serve Performance. *J. Strength Cond. Res. 18(3), 654-656,* Copyright 2004 National Strength & Conditioning Association

72. Duane V. Knudson, Kati Bennet, Rod Corn, David Leick, and Chris Smith. Acute Effects of Stretching are Not Evident in the Kinematics of Vertical Jump. *J. Strength Cond. Res. 15(1), 98-101,* Copyright 2001 National Strength & Conditioning Association

73. Knudson, Duane; Mache, Melissa; Kote, Jessica. Stretching Has No Effect on Free Throw Shooting Accuracy. *Medicine and*

Science in Sports and Exercise: Volume 36(5) Supplement May 2004 p. S206, Copyright 2005 American College of Sports Medicine

74. Kokkonen, J; Allerd, J.. The Effects of Chronic Sports Massage on Strength and Flexibility. *Medicine and Science in Sports and Exercise: Volume 34(5) Supplement 1 May 2002 p. 47,* Copyright 2005 American College of Sports Medicine

75. Kokkonen, Joke; Eldredge, Caroline; Nelson, Arnold G.. Chronic Static Stretching Improves Specific Sports Skills 368. *Medicine and Science in Sports and Exercise: Volume 29(5) Supplement May 1997 p. 63,* Copyright 2005 American College of Sports Medicine

76. Kokkenen, J.; Nelson, A. G.. Acute Stretching Exercises Inhibit Maximal Strength Performance 1130. *Medicine and Science in Sports and Exercise: Volume 28(5) Supplement May 1996 p. 190,* Copyright 2005 American College of Sports Medicine

77. Kravitz, L.. Comparison of Active Assistive to Contract - Relax Stretching. *Medicine and Science in Sports and Exercise: Volume 31(5) Supplement May 1999 p. S115,* Copyright 2005 American College of Sports Medicine

78. Lai K.; O'Kroy, J. A.; Torok, D. J.; Graves, B. S.. Active Isolation Stretching Does Not Improve Hamstring Flexibility Better Than Traditional Stretching Methods. *Medicine and Science in Sports and Exercise: Volume 35)5) Supplement 1 May 2003 p. S79,* Copyright 2005 American College of Sports Medicine

79. LaRoche, Dain P.; Bilodeau, Lindsay; Crowe, Justin; Lynch, Shane. Viscoelastic Response of Skeletal Muscle to Four Days of Flexibility Training. *Medicine and Science in Sports and Exercise: Volume 36(5) Supplement May 2004 p. S345,* Copyright 2005 American College of Sports Medicine

80. Li, Yuhua; Sun, Xusheng; Weiss, Lawrence W.. Hip Joint Abduction Range of Motion During Tai Chi Exercise: 545 Board #136 3:30 PM - 5:00 PM. *Medicine and Science in Sports and Exercise: Volume 37(5) Supplement May 2005 p. S104*, Copyright 2005 American College of Sports Medicine

81. Liemohn, W.; Mazis, N.; Zhang, S. Effect of Active Isolated and Static Stretch Training on Active Straight Leg Raise Performance. *Medicine and Science in Sports and Exercise: Volume 31(5) Supplement May 1999 p. S116*, Copyright 2005 American College of Sports Medicine

82. MacDonncha, C.; McGrath, S.; O'Gorman, D. J.; Warrington, G. D.. The Relationship Between Muscle Flexibility and Sagittal Spinal Posture in Gaelic Football Players. *Medicine and Science in Sports and Exercise: Volume 35(5) Supplement 1 May 2003 p. S191*, Copyright 2005 American College of Sports Medicine

83. Magnusson, S. P.; Larsson, B.. Altered Hamstring Flexibility, Stiffness and Stretch Tolerance in Runners 391. *Medicine and Science in Sports and Exercise: Volume 29(5) Supplement May 1997 p. 68*, Copyright 2005 American College of Sports Medicine

84. Magnusson, S. P.; Aaagaard, P.; Simonsen, E. Hamstring Flexibility and Muscle Stiffness. *Medicine and Science in Sports and Exercise: Volume 36(5) Supplement May 1998 p. 115*, Copyright 2005 American College of Sports Medicine

85. Magnusson, P.; Simonsen, E.; Aagaard, P.; Klinge, K.; Kjaer, M.. Flexibility and Resistance to Stretch 385. *Medicine and Science in Sports and Exercise: Volume 28(5) Supplement May 1996 p. 65*, Copyright 2005 American College of Sports Medicine

86. Magnusson, S. P.; Aagaard, P.; Neilson J. Juul.. Energy Return After Stretch. *Medicine and Science in Sports and Exercise: Volume*

31(5) Supplement May 1999 p. S276, Copyright 2005 American College of Sports Medicine

87. Nikos Malliaropoulus, Stelios Papalezandris, Agape Papalada, and Emanuel Papacostas. The Role of Stretching in 'Rehabilitation of Hamstring Injuries: 80 Athletes Follow-Up. *Medicine and Science in Sports and Exercise: Volume 36(5) p. 756-759, 2004* Copyright 2005 American College of Sports Medicine

88. Manire, John T.; Adams, Kent J.; Swank, Ann M.; Kipp, Robert L.; Stamford, Bryant, A.. Diurnal Variation of Hamstring and Lumbar Flexibility. *Medicine and Science in Sports and Exercise: Volume 36(5) Supplement May 2004 p. S356,* Copyright 2005 American College of Sports Medicine

89. Marino, J.; Ramsey, J. M.; Otto, R. M.; Wygand, J. W.. The Effects of Active Isolated Vs Static Stretching on Flexibility. Manire, John T.; Adams, Kent J.; Swank, Ann M.; Kipp, Robert L.; Stamford, Bryant, A.. Diurnal Variation of Hamstring and Lumbar Flexibility. *Medicine and Science in Sports and Exercise: Volume 36(5) Supplement May 2004 p. S356,* Copyright 2005 American College of Sports Medicine

90. Mastrangelo, M. A.; Galantino, Mary Lou; Chaluopka, Edward C.. Effects of Yoga on Quility Of Life and Flexibility In Perimenopausal and Postmenopausal Women:420 Board#11 2:00 PM -3:30 PM. *Medicine and Science in Sports and Exercise: Volume 37(5) Supplement May 2005 p. S75,* Copyright 2005 American College of Sports Medicine

91. McHugh, Malachy P.; Kremenic, Ian J.; Fox, Michael B.; Gleim, Gilbert W.. The Role of Mechanical and Neural Restraints to Joint Range of Motion During Passive Stretch. *Medicine and Science in Sports and Exercise: Volume 30(6) p. 928-932, June 1998,* Copyright 2005 American College of Sports Medicine

92. Peter J. McNair, Erik W. Dombroski, David J. Hewson, and Stephen N. Stanley. Stretching at the Ankle Joint; Viscoelastic Responses to Holds and Continuous Passive Motion. *Medicine and Science in Sports and Exercise: Volume 33(3) 2000 pp. 354-358,* Copyright 2005 American College of Sports Medicine

93. Mello, Monica L.; Pereira, Marta; Gomes, Paulo Sergio Chagas. Acute Effect of Static and PNF Stretching ON Dominant Knee Flexion and Extension Strength: 951 Board #173 10:30 AM - 12:00 PM. *Medicine and Science in Sports and Exercise: Volume 33(5) Supplement 1 May 2001 p. S10,* Copyright 2005 American College of Sports Medicine

94. McHugh, Malachy P.; Kremenic, Ian J.; Fox, Michael B.; Gleim, Gilbert W.. The Role of Mechanical and Neural Restraints to Joint Range of Motion During Passive Stretch. *Medicine and Science in Sports and Exercise: Volume 30(6) p. 928-932, June 1998,* Copyright 2005 American College of Sports Medicine

95. Mello, Monica L.; Pereira, Marta; Gomes, Paulo Sergio Chagas. Acute Effect of Static and PNF Stretching ON Dominant Knee Flexion and Extension Strength: 951 Board #173 10:30 AM - 12:00 PM. *Medicine and Science in Sports and Exercise: Volume 37(5) Supplement May 2005 p. S183,* Copyright 2005 American College of Sports Medicine

96. Messner, B.; Guyer, S.; Holder, J.; Skelton, M. Effect of Plyometric Training on Strength, Vertical Jump, Flexibility and Range of Motion in Volleyball Players. *Medicine and Science in Sports and Exercise: Volume 31(5) Supplement May 1999 p. S281,* Copyright 2005 American College of Sports Medicine

97. Middag, T. R.; Harmer P. Active Isolated Stretching is Not More Effective Than Static Stretching for Increasing Hamstring Flexibility. *Medicine and Science in Sports and Exercise: Volume*

34(5) Supplement 1 May 2002 p. S151, Copyright 2005 American College of Sports Medicine

98. Alan E. Mikesky, Rafael E. Bahamonde, Katie Staton, Thurman Alvey, and Tom Fitton. Acute Effects of The Stick on Strength, Power, and Flexibility. *J. Strength Cond. Res. 16(3), 446-450,* Copyright 2002 National Strength & Conditioning Association

99. Millar, A.L.; Raasch, P.; Robinson, Y.; St. Jean, G.; Wolff, C. F.; Perry, W.L.. Hamstring Flexibility of Pre Pubertal Through Post Pubertal Individuals. *Medicine and Science in Sports and Exercise: Volume 33(5) Supplement 1 May 2001 p. S10,* Copyright 2005 American College of Sports Medicine

100. Miller, Doug K.; Kieffer, Scott, Hansen-Kieffer, Kris; Ken Heck. Changes I Hamstring Flexibility Following Supervised and Unsupervised Stretching Programs. *Medicine and Science in Sports and Exercise: Volume 36(5) Supplement May 2004 p. S356,* Copyright 2005 American College of Sports Medicine

101. Miyahara, Yutestu; Ogura, Yuji; Naito, Hisashi; Katamoto, Shizuo; Aoki, Junichiro. Effect of Proprioceptive Neuromuscular Facilitation Stretching and Static Stretching on Maximal Voluntary Contraction: 2281 Board#70 10:30 AM - 12:00 PM. *Medicine and Science in Sports and Exercise: Volume 37(5) Supplement May 2005 p. S441,* Copyright 2005 American College of Sports Medicine

102. Swapan Mookeerjee, Khalid W. Bibi, Gregory A. Kenney, and Lee Cohen. Relationship Between Isokinetic Strength, Flexibility, and Flutter Kicking Speed in Female Collegiate Swimmers. *J. Strength Cond. Res. 9(2), 71-74,* Copyright 1995 National Strength & Conditioning Association

103. Nelson, A.G.; Cornwell, A.; Heise, G. D.. Acute Stretching Exercises and Vertical Jump Stored Elastic Energy927. *Medicine and Science*

in Sports and Exercise: Volume 28(5) Supplement May 1996 p. 156, Copyright 2005 American College of Sports Medicine

104. Arnold G. Nelson, Ivan K. Guillory, Andrew Cornwell, and Joke Kokkenen. Inhibition of Maximal Voluntary Isokinetic Torque Production Following Stretching is Velocity Specific. *J. Strength Cond. Res. 15(2), 241-246*, Copyright 2001 National Strength & Conditioning Association

105. Nelson, Arnold G.; Kokkonen, Joke; de Leon, Miguel; Koeber, Garret; Nishime, Miwa; Smith, Joshua. Passive Static Stretching Elevates Heart Rate During Subsequent Moderately High Intensity Cycling. *Medicine and Science in Sports and Exercise: Volume 36(5) Supplement May 2004 p. S356*, Copyright 2005 American College of Sports Medicine

106. Nelson, Arnold G.; Kokkonen, Joke; de Leon, Miguel; Koeber, Garret; Nishime, Miwa; Smith, Joshua. Passive Static Stretching Elevates Metabolic Rates: 544 Board #135 2:00 PM - 3:30 PM. *Medicine and Science in Sports and Exercise: Volume 37(5) Supplement May 2005 p. S103-S104*, Copyright 2005 American College of Sports Medicine

107. Nelson, A.G.; Kokkonen, J.; Arnall, D.A.; Kalani, W.; Peterson, K.; Kenly, M.. A Ten Week Stretching Program Increases Strength in the Contralateral Muscle. *Medicine and Science in Sports and Exercise: Volume 34(5) Supplement 1 May 2002 p. S287*, Copyright 2005 American College of Sports Medicine

108. Arnold G. Nelson, Joke Kokkonen, and David A. Arnall. Acute Muscle Stretching Inhibits Muscle Strength Endurance Performance. *J. Strength Cond. Res. 19(2), 338-343*, Copyright 2005 National Strength & Conditioning Association

109. Nelson, A. G.; Kokkonen, J.; Eldredge, C.; Cornwell, A.; Glickman-Weiss, E. Chronic Stretching and Running Economy 394. *Medicine*

and Science in Sports and Exercise: Volume 29(5) Supplement May 1997 p. 68, Copyright 2005 American College of Sports Medicine

110. Noffal, GuillermoJ.; Knudson, Duane; Brown, Lee. Effects of Stretching on Throwing Speed and Isokinetic Shoulder Torques. *Medicine and Science in Sports and Exercise: Volume 36(5) Supplement May 2004 p. S136-137,* Copyright 2005 American College of Sports Medicine

111. O'Connor, J.S., Hines K.; Warner. C.A.. Flexibility and Injury Incidence 376. *Medicine and Science in Sports and Exercise: Volume 28(5) Supplement May 1996 p. 63,* Copyright 2005 American College of Sports Medicine

112. Paula, K. C.; Carvalho, A. C. G.; Azevedo, T. M. C.; Nobrega, A. C. L.. Interaction Between Resistance and Flexibility Training in Healthy Young Adults. *Medicine and Science in Sports and Exercise: Volume 30(5) Supplement May 1998 p. S200,* Copyright 2005 American College of Sports Medicine

113. Patrick C. Sawyer, Tim L. Uhl, Carl G. Mattacola, Darren L. Johnson, and James W. Yates. Effects of Moist Heat on Hamstring Flexibility and Muscle Temperature. *J. Strength Cond. Res. 17(2), 285-290,* Copyright 2003 National Strength & Conditioning Association

114. Rodney Peter Pope, Robert Dale Herbert, John Dennis Kirwan, and Bruce James Graham. A Randomized Trial of Preexercise Stretching for Prevention of Lower-limb Injury. *Medicine and Science in Sports and Exercise: Volume 32(2) p. 271-277, 2000,* Copyright 2005 American College of Sports Medicine

115. Kevin Power, David Behm, Farrel Cahill, Michael Carrol, and Warren Young. An Acute Bout of Static Stretching: Effects on Force and Jumping Performance. *Medicine and Science in Sports and Exercise: Volume 36(8) p. 1389-1396, 2004* Copyright 2005 American College of Sports Medicine

116. 116. Puhl, J. J.; Perry, A.; Signorile, J.F.; Miller, P.C.. The Effects of A Flexibility Program on Low Back Pain 48. *Medicine and Science in Sports and Exercise: Volume 28(5) Supplement 1 May 1996 p. 8*, Copyright 2005 American College of Sports Medicine

117. Duncan A. Reid and Peter J. McNair. Passive Force, Angle, and Stiffness Changes after Stretching of Hamstring Muscles. *Medicine and Science in Sports and Exercise: Volume 36(11) p. 1944-1948, 2004* Copyright 2005 American College of Sports Medicine

118. E. Paul Roetert, Todd S. Ellenbecker, and Scott W. Brown. Shoulder Internal and External Rotation Range of Motion in Nationally Ranked Junior Tennis Players: A Longitudinal Analysis. *J. Strength Cond. Res. 14(2), 140-143*, Copyright 2000 National Strength & Conditioning Association

119. Michael Ross. Effect of Lower -Extremity Position and Stretching on Hamstring Muscle Flexibility. *J. Strength Cond. Res. 13(2), 124-129*, Copyright 1999 National Strength & Conditioning Association

120. Rubinfeld, M. J.; Wygand, J.; Otto, R. M.. Hamstring Flexibility as Assessed by Multiple Angle Sit and Reach Box Apparatus. *Medicine and Science in Sports and Exercise: Volume 34(5) Supplement 1 May 2002 p. S151*, Copyright 2005 American College of Sports Medicine

121. Rubini, Ercole D.; Pereira, Marta; Gomez, Paulo Sergio C.. Acute Effect of Static Stretching and PNF Stretching on Hip Adductor Isometric Strength: 953 Board #175 10: 30 AM - 12:00 PM. *Medicine and Science in Sports and Exercise: Volume 37(5) Supplement May 2005 p. S183-184*, Copyright 2005 American College of Sports Medicine

122. Sato, H.; Sato, M.; Kan, A.; Goto, N.; Masuda, S.; Fukuba, Y. Relations Between Lower Leg Musculature, Flexibility, and Mobility Status

in Extremely Old-Aged Women. *Medicine and Science in Sports and Exercise: Volume 33(5) Supplement 1 May 2001 p. S118,* Copyright 2005 American College of Sports Medicine

123. Schwellnus, M. P.; Cobbing, S.; Noakes, T. D.. Proprioceptive Neuromuscular Facilitation (PNF) Stretching: What is the Optimum Duration, Type, and Frequency. *Medicine and Science in Sports and Exercise: Volume 33(5) Supplement 1 May 2001 p. S197,* Copyright 2005 American College of Sports Medicine

124. Scott, Sue M.; Rosenberg, Rachel I.. Methods To Improve and Maintain Balance, Mobility, Flexibility and Balance Confidence in Older Individuals: 1316 Board #171000 3:30 PM - 5:00 PM. *Medicine and Science in Sports and Exercise: Volume 37(5) Supplement May 2005 p. S256,* Copyright 2005 American College of Sports Medicine

125. Serrano, Ronnie; Russo, Anne Marie; Marino Joseph; Lamonte, Alyson; Wygand, John; Otto Robert M. A Comparison of the Traditional Vs The Unilateral Back Saver Sit and Reach Hamstring Stretch: 490 Board #81 2:00 PM - 3:30 PM. *Medicine and Science in Sports and Exercise: Volume 37(5) Supplement May 2005 p. S92,* Copyright 2005 American College of Sports Medicine

126. Guy G. Simoneau. The Impact of Various Anthropometric and Flexibility Measurements on the Sit-and-Reach Test. *J. Strength Cond. Res. 12(4), 232-237,* Copyright 1998 National Strength & Conditioning Association

127. Simonson, S. R.. Longer Duration Circuit Training Improves Flexibility and Strength in College Men and Women. *Medicine and Science in Sports and Exercise: Volume 35(5) Supplement 1 May 2003 p. S402,* Copyright 2005 American College of Sports Medicine

128. Spencer, S. J.; Cornelius, W. L.; Hill, D. W.. Concentric and Isometric Actions in Proprioceptive Neuromuscular Facilitation Stretching Techniques. *Medicine and Science in Sports and Exercise: Volume 30(5) Supplement May 1998 p. 164*, Copyright 2005 American College of Sports Medicine

129. Stephen B. Thacker, Julie Gilchrist, Donna F. Stroup, and C. Dexter Kimsey, Jr.. The Impact of Stretching of Sports Injury Risk: A Systematic Review of the Literature. *Medicine and Science in Sports and Exercise: Volume 36(3) p. 371-378, 2004*, Copyright 2005 American College of Sports Medicine

130. Ann Marie Swank, Daniel C. Funk, Michael P. Durham, and Sherri Roberts. Adding Weights to Stretching Exercises Increases Passive Range of Motion for Healthy Adults. *J. Strength Cond. Res. 17(2), 374-378*, Copyright 2003 National Strength & Conditioning Association

131. Swank, S. A.; Long, K. A.; Lee, E. J.; Poindexter, H. B.. Strength, Flexibility, and Body Composition Changes of Older Women Following 10 Weeks of Water Exercise. *Medicine and Science in Sports and Exercise: Volume 28(5) Supplement May 1996 p. 189*, Copyright 2005 American College of Sports Medicine

132. Kevin Thrash and Brian Kelly. Research Notes: Flexibility and Strength Training. *Journal of Applied Sport Science Research 1(4) p. 74-75, 1987*, Copyright National Strength and Conditioning Association

133. Jessica Unick, H. Scott Kieffer, Wendy Cheesman, and Anna Feeney. The Acute Effects of Static and Ballistic Stretching on Vertical Jump Performance in Trained Women. *J. Strength Cond. Res. 19(1), 206-212*, Copyright 2005 National Strength & Conditioning Association

134. Valim-Rogatto, Priscila C.; Rogatto, Gustavo P. Interference of Stretching and Music on Stress Symptoms of Brazilian Pre-University Students. *Medicine and Science in Sports and Exercise: Volume 36(5) Supplement May 2004 p. S355-S356*, Copyright 2005 American College of Sports Medicine

135. Harvey W. Wallman, John A. Mercer, and J. Wesley McWhorter Surface Electromyographic Assessment of the Effect of Static Stretching of the Gastronomies on Vertical Jump Performance. *J. Strength Cond. Res. 19(3), 684-688*, Copyright 2005 National Strength & Conditioning Association

136. Weiss S.; Hsaio, D.; Wygard, J.; Otto, R.M.. The Effects of Passive Stretching on Performance During Delayed Onset Muscle Soreness . *Medicine and Science in Sports and Exercise: Volume 31(5) Supplement May 1999 p. S208*, Copyright 2005 American College of Sports Medicine

137. David L. Wenos and Jeff G. Konin. Controlled Warm-UP Intensity Enhances Hip Range of Motion. *J. Strength Cond. Res. 18(3), 529-533*, Copyright 2004 National Strength & Conditioning Association

138. Williams, Valerie; Lynn, Jeff; Pierce, Patricia. How Flexible are The Flexibility Tests? A Comparison Using Ultramarathon Runners: 517 Board #108 3:30 PM - 5:00 PM. *Medicine and Science in Sports and Exercise: Volume 37(5) Supplement May 2005 p. S98*, Copyright 2005 American College of Sports Medicine

139. Wittmann, Marie; Babault, Nicolas; Kouassi, Blah Y. L.. Static Stretch and Warm -Up: Effects On The Lower Limb Flexibility and Jumping Ability: 991 Board #213 10:30 AM - 12:00 PM. *Medicine and Science in Sports and Exercise: Volume Supplement May p. ,* Copyright 2005 American College of Sports Medicine

140. Woolstenhulme, Mandy; Multer, Christine E.; Woolenstenhulme, Emily; Parcell, Allen C.. Ballistic Stretching Increases Flexibility and Acute Vertical Jump Height When Combined with Basketball Activity. *Medicine and Science in Sports and Exercise: Volume 36(5) Supplement May 2004 p. S346-S347*, Copyright 2005 American College of Sports Medicine

141. Ian C. Wright, Richard R. Neptune, Anton J. Van Den Bogert, and Benno M. Nigg. The Effects of Ankle Compliance and Flexibility on Ankle Sprains. *Medicine and Science in Sports and Exercise: Volume 32(3) p. 260-265, 2000*, Copyright 2005 American College of Sports Medicine

142. Taichi Yamguchi and Kojiro Ishii. Effects of Static Stretching for 30 Seconds and Dynamic Stretching on Leg Extension Power. *J. Strength Cond. Res. 19(3), 677-683*, Copyright 2005 National Strength & Conditioning Association

143. Yarrow, Joshua F.; Burns, Trevor W.. Static Stretching Inhibits Maximal Muscle Endurance. *Medicine and Science in Sports and Exercise: Volume 36(5) Supplement May 2004 p. S353*, Copyright 2005 American College of Sports Medicine

Bibliography:
Chapter Section 3: Chapter 9

1. Annesi JJ. *Goal-Setting Protocol in Adherence to Exercise by Italian Adults. Percept Mot Skills. 2002 Apr;94(2):453-8.*, PMID 12027338 [PubMed - indexed for MEDLINE]

2. Anthony J.. Psychologic Aspects of Exercise. *Clin Sports Med. 1991 Jan; 10(1): 171-80.*, PMID 2015642 [PubMed - indexed for MEDLINE]

3. Thomas R. Baechle, Roger W. Earle. Essentials of Strength Training and Conditioning - 2nd Edition. Pgs. 194-201, 251-255, Copyright 2000, 1994 National Strength and Condition Association.

4. Siri Carpenter. *They're positively inspiring.* Monitor on Psychology Volume 32, No. 7 July/August 2001

5. Chervak, M Canham; Knapik, J J.; Hauret, K G.; Arnold, S; Hoedebecke, E L. Lee, R B.. Application of the Intrinsic Inventory in U.S. Army Basic Training. *Medicine & Science in Sports & Exercise May 2003, 35:5 Supplement 1 p S149,* Copyright American College of Sports Medicine 2004

6. Michael A. Clark, Rodney J. Corn. NASM OPT Optimum Performance Training for the Fitness Professional, 2nd Edition. Copyright 2001, National Academy of Sports Medicine. pg. 297, 301, 315, 375-377, 434, 438

7. Scott L. Cresswell, Robert C. Eklund. Motivation and Burnout among Top Amateur Rugby Players. *Medicine & Science in Sports & Exercise Volume 37, No. 3, pp. 469-477, 2005,* Copyright American College of Sports Medicine 2005

8. De Bourdeaudhuij. Lefevre, Philippaerts, Matton, Wijndaele, *Validity and Usefulness of Stages of Change For Physical Activity in a Representative Adolescent Sample,* Medicine & Science in Sports &

9. Edward L. Deci and Richard M. Ryan. The "What" and Why of Goal Pursuits: Human Needs and the Self Determination of Behavior. *Psychological Inquiry 2000, Vol. 11, No. 4, 227-268*

10. 10. Divine, J.; Chorley, j.; Kohl, h,; Cianca, j.. Motivation for Starting Marathon Training Program: Running Experience and Gender Differences. Medicine & Science in Sports & Exercise:

Volume31(5) Supplement May 1999 p. S93, Copyright Lippincott Williams & Wilkins, Inc.

11. Epstein, Leonard H.; Roemmich, James N. Reducing Sedentary Behavior: Role in Modifying Physical Activity, *Exercise and Sports Science Review: Volume 29(3) July 2001 pp 103-108,* Copyright American College of Sports Medicine 2004

12. Gauvin L. An Experiential Perspective on the Motivational Features of Exercise and Lifestyle
Can J Sport Sci. 1990 Mar; 15(1): 7-8, PMID 2331640 [PubMed - indexed for MEDLINE]

13. Godin G., Shephard RJ. Use of Attitude-Behavior Models in Exercise Promotion
Sports Med. 1990 Aug; 10(2): 103-21, PMID 2204097 [PubMed - indexed for MEDLINE]

14. Stephen C. Glass, Douglas R. Stanton. Self-Selected Resistance Training Intensity in Novice Weightlifters, *J. Strength Cond. Res., 2004, 18(2), 324-327,* Copyright 2004 National Strength and Conditioning Association

15. Hamp, E K.; Faghre, P D.; Sheehan, N W.; Armstrong, L E.; Bohannon, R. W.. Exercise Adherence in Older Adults: A Behavior Modification Approach. *Medicine & Science in Sports & Exercise May 2003, 35:5 Supplement 1 p S74,* Copyright American College of Sports Medicine 2004

16. Hills, A. P.; Byrne, N. M.. Body Composition, Body Satisfaction and Exercise Motivation of Girls and Boys. *Medicine & Science in Sports & Exercise: Volume30(5) Supplement May 1998 p. S120,* Copyright Lippincott Williams & Wilkins, Inc.

17. Elizabeth Howell. Motivation Therapy. Medscape / Copyright 2004 Medscape

18. Edward T. Howley, B. Don Franks. Health Fitness Instructors Handbook - 3rd Edition. pg. 196-197, 232-233, 304, 306. Human Kinetics, Copyright 1997, 1992, 1986 by Edward T. Howley and B. Don Franks

19. Kerner MS, Grossman AH. Attitudinal, Social, and Practical Correlates to Fitness Behaviour: A Test of the Theory of Planned Behaviour. *Percept Mot Skills. 1998 Dec;87(3pt 2): 1139-54*, PMID 10052071 [PubMed - indexed for MEDLINE]

20. Kilpatrick, M., Bartholomew, J., Hebert, E.. Behavioral Regulations in Physical Activity: A Comparison of Sport and Exercise Motivation, *Medicine & Science in Sports & Exercise May 2003, 35:5 Supplement 1 p S150,* Copyright American College of Sports Medicine 2004

21. Lee, R E.; DiClemente, C C. Extrinsic and Intrinsic Motivation: Which Is Important for Exercise. *Medicine & Science in Sports & Exercise: Volume33(5) Supplement May 2001 p. S113,* Copyright 2001 American College of Sports Medicine

22. Bess H. Marcus, Beth A. Lewis. Physical Activity and The Stages of Motivational Readiness for Change Model. *Research Digest, Series 4, No. 1, March 2003,* Presidents Counsel of Physical Fitness and Sports

23. Steven R. McClaran. The Effectiveness of Personal Training on Changing Attitudes Towards Physical Activity. *JSSM 2003 - 2, 10- 14,* Copyright 2003 Journal of Sports Science and Medicine

24. Patrick J. O' Connor and Timothy W. Puetz. Chronic Physical Activity and Feelings of Energy and Fatigue. *Medicine & Science in Sports & Exercise: Volume 37 No. 2 pp. 299-305. 2005,* Copyright 2005 American College of Sports Medicine

25. Rhodes, Courneya. Threshold Assessment of The Theory of Planned Behaviour for Predicting Exercise Intention and Behaviour, *Medicine & Science in Sports & Exercise, 35:5 Supplement 1 May 2003 p S149*, Copyright American College of Sports Medicine 2004

26. Rhodes, R. E.; Jones, L. W.; Courneya, K.S.. Moderating Effects of Personality on Exercise Motivation. *Medicine & Science in Sports & Exercise 33:5 Supplement 1 May 2001 p S64*, Copyright American College of Sports Medicine 2001

27. Schnider, Lee Buckworth; DiClemente. Intrinsic and Extrinsic Motivation and Stage of Exercise Adoption: Results from Two Samples, *Medicine & Science in Sports & Exercise May 2003, 35:5 Supplement 1 p S149*, Copyright American College of Sports Medicine 2004

28. Serfass RC, Gerberich SG. Exercise for Optimal Health: Strategies and Motivational Considerations, *Prev. Med. 1984 Jan;13(1):79-99*, PMID 6371780 [PubMed - indexed for MEDLINE]

29. Siegel, S R.; Pena Reyes, M E.; Cardenas Barahona, E E.; Malina, R M.. Motivation For Sport and for Discontinuing Sport in Normal Weight and Overweight Mexican Youth. *Medicine & Science in Sports & Exercise: Volume33(5) Supplement May 2001 p. S113*, Copyright 2001 American College of Sports Medicine

30. Smith R. A.; Biddle S. J.. Attitudes and Exercise Adherence: Test of Theories of Reasoned Action And Planned Behaviour. *J Sports Sci. 1990 Apr:17(4):269-81.*, PMID 10373037 [PubMed - indexed for MEDLINE]

31. Stewart, C. C.; Meyers, M. C. Motivation and Locus of Control of Elite, Teenage Soccer Players. *Medicine & Science in Sports &*

Exercise: Volume31(5) Supplement May 1999 p. S217, Copyright Lippincott Williams & Wilkins, Inc.

32. William R. Sukala. Master of Science Degree Thesis: Nutrition Knowledge and Information Sources of Active Individuals. San Diego State University, Department of Exercise and Nutritional Sciences

33. A Report of The Surgeon General. Physical Activity and Health: Adults. *U.S Departments of Health and Human Services: National Center for Chronic Disease Prevention and Health Promotion, Center of Disease Control and Prevention(CDC), The Presidents Council on Physical Fitness and Sports*

34. Gershon Tenebaum, Howard K. Hall, Nick Calcagnini, Rael Lange, Gavin Freeman, Michael Loyd*Coping With Physical Exertion and Negative Feedback Under Competitive and Self-Standard Conditions*Journal of Applied Psychology, 2001, 31, 8, pp. 1582-1626 Copyright 2001 by V. H. Winston & Son, Inc.

35. Piotr Unierzyski, PhD. Level of Achievement Motivation of Young Tennis Players and Their Future Progress. *J. Sports Sci. & Med. (2003) 2, 184-186*, Copyright 2003 Journal of Sports Science and Medicine

36. Warren, B.; Newton M.; Niedfeldt, C.. Relationship of Psychological, Anatomical and Achievement Motivation Goals to Injury Conditions in Professional Soccer Players. *Medicine & Science in Sports & Exercise May 2003, 35:5 Supplement 1 p S150*, Copyright American College of Sports Medicine 2004

37. Whaley, D E.; Schnider, A F.. The Effects of A Structured, Individualized Exercise Program on the Motivation of Older Adult Exercisers. *Medicine & Science in Sports & Exercise: Volume33(5) Supplement May 2001 p. S112*, Copyright 2001 American College of Sports Medicine

CPSIA information can be obtained
at www.ICGtesting.com
Printed in the USA
FFOW04n1315010916
27340FF